THE CHIROPRACTOR'S HEALTH BOOK

THE CHIROPRACTOR'S HEALTH BOOK

simple, natural exercises for relieving
headaches, tension, and back pain

DR. LEONARD McGILL

THREE RIVERS PRESS
NEW YORK

Grateful acknowledgment is made to the following for permission to reprint illustrations and photographs: Krames Communications, a K-III Education Company for the illustrations on pages 42, 43, and 69. Avia Athletic Footwear for the photographs on page 138. Dupont for the photograph on page 139. Coffee cartoon on p. 50, copyright 1991, by Lee Michielle, *The New Yorker*. Hilda Muinos for the original illustrations on pages 18, 66, and 96.

Published by Three Rivers Press, a division of Crown Publishers, Inc., 201 East 50th Street, New York, New York 10022. Member of the Crown Publishing Group.

Random House, Inc. New York, Toronto, London, Sydney, Auckland
http://www.randomhouse.com/

THREE RIVERS PRESS and colophon are trademarks of Crown Publishers, Inc.

Printed in the United States of America

Design by Maggie Hinders

Library of Congress Cataloging-in-Publication Data
McGill, Leonard.
  The chiropractor's health book / by Leonard McGill.
  Includes index.
  1. Chiropractic—Popular works. I. Title.
RZ244.M38   1997   615.5'34—dc20   96–23966

ISBN 0-517-88818-1

10 9 8 7 6 5

Dedicated to my loving wife
and gifted chiropractor
DR. JEANNE-MARIE KANE

CONTENTS

ACKNOWLEDGMENTS

Thanks to all my chiropractic colleagues past and present, who are working so hard to develop the greatest healing art in the world.

Special thanks to those who've shared their philosophy and clinical knowledge with me, including Dr. Harvey Fish, Dr. Jerry Hochman, Dr. Will May, Dr. Kevin Millet, Dr. Steve Taylor, Dr. Sid Williams, and Dr. Reggie Gold.

I'm grateful to my staff at Life Chiropractic Center in Salt Lake City, Utah, including Anthony Simone and Heather Hutchings, for their help in researching and preparing this book. Also, many thanks to my fantastic editor, Eliza Scott, and to Connie and Lisa at Connie Clausen Associates, for their support.

It's with great love and appreciation that I extend the warmest thanks to all my patients at Life Chiropractic Center, without whom this book would not have been possible.

THE
CHIROPRACTOR'S
HEALTH
BOOK

INTRODUCTION

Perhaps like you, throughout my youth I took good health for granted. Maybe you remember when your body first gave you signs you weren't always going to be invincible. For me that happened while attending college in 1977, when my neck started hurting. I took aspirin but it didn't work, so I went to the infirmary and the doctor gave me some stronger pills. They didn't work either, and throughout my senior year my neck pain kept getting worse.

After college I went to New York to write for magazines, and my neck started torturing me with a vengeance, producing headaches that would start at the base of my skull and travel to behind my eyes.

The neck pain and headaches became a curse. For example, once, in the early eighties, while working for *GQ*, the men's lifestyle/fashion magazine, I went to interview Valentino. I'd never seen anything as grand as the Italian fashion designer's penthouse apartment. He'd hosted a birthday party for Jackie Onassis earlier in the day. Hundreds of fresh carnations and roses in bouquets the size of beach balls bloomed from the living room's every tabletop. It could have been a magical moment, but as I waited to talk with one of the most influential designers of the twentieth century, I became depressed; all I could think about was how badly my neck hurt.

At that time I was using a lot of a particularly hellish liniment formulated to relieve "sore, aching muscles." This product is still very popular. It's greasy and smelly and comes in a plastic tub. When you first rub it on your skin it's subzero cold, then it turns so hot it feels like someone's searing you with a blowtorch. I'd buy jumbo-size containers of this product and keep them on my bathroom sink, smearing globs on the back of my neck in order to sleep at night. It wasn't very romantic.

The headaches kept getting worse, and I started going from doctor to doctor, trying different medications, undergoing different tests. Finally, my family physician said, "Mr. McGill, you need a psychiatrist; you're obviously generating these neck pains and headaches in your mind." So he sent me to a shrink. I didn't know it at the time, but it happened to be his brother-in-law.

The psychiatrist charged me eighty dollars twice a week for my fifty-minute sessions, and prescribed Xanax and Valium, two powerful tranquilizers. Within six weeks I became addicted. I also became nearly impotent and totally lethargic. At one o'clock in the afternoon I could lay my head on my desk and be out cold for hours at a time—*and neck pains and headaches were still making my life miserable!* (Though, thanks to my psychiatric sessions, I was learning that somehow Mighty Mouse had played a large part in my early development.)

At about this time I met a woman who said, "You need to see my chiropractor, Dr. Harvey Fish." Dr. Fish practiced on West 72nd Street. I went to see him and he explained that two automobile accidents and several football injuries had left my neck with more kinks than a flight of stairs. Bones were misaligned, pinching on nerves. He went to work, and within two months my headaches and neck pain vanished. I threw away the pills, began sleeping through the night, lost weight, became more energetic than I'd been in five years, and said, "Wow! This stuff is so great I have to become a chiropractor!"

That's how I got here, writing a book for you.

Chiropractic never crossed my mind before my friend told me about Dr. Fish, but it's been making sick people well for more than a hundred

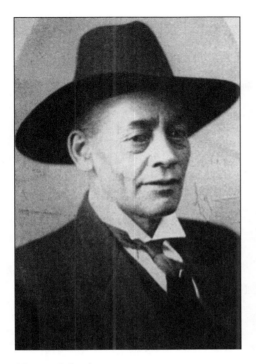 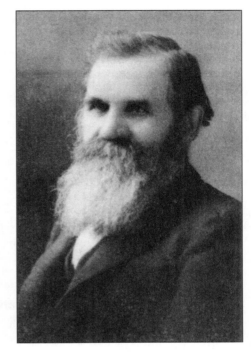

Harvey Lillard.   D. D. Palmer.

years. Most people associate chiropractors with relieving back pain, neck pain, and headaches, but it started by helping people with much more serious problems.

It was September 18, 1895, in Davenport, Iowa. Harvey Lillard, who was deaf, was working as a janitor, cleaning out the office of Dr. D. D. Palmer. Palmer knew Lillard hadn't always been deaf, because the man could speak. The doctor wrote Lillard a note on a slip of paper, inquiring how he'd lost his hearing. Lillard said he'd been working in a stooped position one day when something "gave" in his back. Soon afterward his hearing had faded.

Palmer asked the janitor if he might examine him and Lillard agreed, lying down on a bench. A large lump could be seen on his neck. It appeared that a bone there was misaligned.

Palmer received permission to try putting the bone back into its proper position. Placing his hands on the spine, the doctor gave a forceful thrust. There was a loud pop.

It was a hot day in Davenport, and the windows were open. Lillard got off the table. His eyes grew wide as he went to the windows and leaned out. "Dr. Palmer!" he cried. "I can hear the wagon wheels on the cobblestones!" With one spinal adjustment, Lillard recovered his hearing.

Initially, Palmer thought he'd discovered a cure for deafness, but soon realized he was onto something bigger.

"Shortly after this relief from deafness, I had a case of heart trouble which was not improving," Palmer wrote. "I examined the spine and found a displaced vertebra pressing against the nerves which innervate [go to] the heart. I adjusted the vertebra and gave immediate relief. Then I began to reason if two diseases, so dissimilar as deafness and heart trouble, came from impingement, a pressure on nerves, were not other diseases due to a similar cause?"

Palmer began developing his "hand treatments," and was soon getting results with many different conditions. Asthma, colic, ear infections, digestion problems, headaches—virtually any ailment—might be a candidate for the new healing art. Soon people from all over the country were traveling to Davenport for spinal adjustments.

Reverend Samuel Weed, one of Palmer's first patients, gave the new profession a name. He took the Greek word for hand—*cheir*—and "done by"—*praktos*—combining them into *chiropractic*, meaning "done by hand."

Palmer went on to found the Palmer School of Chiropractic in Davenport, and the profession grew quickly. Today there are more than fifty thousand chiropractors in the United States alone. Twenty-six colleges worldwide graduate thousands of spinal experts each year, making chiropractic the fastest-growing health-care profession in the world. According to *Time* magazine, one out of twenty people in the United States will visit a chiropractor this year, and this number is expected to double in the next ten years.

Chiropractic is growing so fast because it *works*. And people are realizing that drugs and surgery, while necessary at times, are not the best way to get or stay healthy. As one of my friends says, "If drugs are so dangerous to take when you're pregnant, why do doctors want to give them to our children?" Another likes to ask his patients who are considering surgery, "Have you ever cut anything that made it more whole?"

Ask yourself, "Do I want more drugs and surgeries in my life?" Most people answer no, realizing that medical intervention only attempts to fix illness. I often pose this question to patients: Can you imagine walking into your local emergency room and saying, "Listen, I feel fantastic today and I want to feel better. Check me in!"?

Medicine's focus on treating problems keeps it from being a tool we can use to attain total wellness and peak performance. In my clinic, if a "healthy" person comes in and wants to get healthier, I can virtually guarantee that person that under chiropractic care he or she will experience more energy, better digestion, better sleep, increased athletic performance, and fewer colds and other health problems.

A chiropractor shared this story with me recently: His mother-in-law died after a six-week stay in a major hospital's intensive care unit. Several "heroic" surgeries were attempted to save the woman's life, to no avail. Her bill for six weeks in the hospital: $400,000.

The chiropractor said, "What if my mother-in-law had taken $400,000 when she was twenty-one and invested it in her health? What if she'd joined the best health club, eaten the most wholesome foods, and paid a good chiropractor to keep her body in top shape? Do you realize it would be nearly impossible to spend $400,000 in your lifetime on staying healthy, and yet you can spend it in six weeks on being sick!"

I believe one of our biggest problems in health care is that we're spending huge amounts treating sickness and disease instead of promoting health within ourselves. There's a sign on the wall in my office reading, "It's better to help the good than fight the bad." After decades of our "war" on cancer, we have higher rates for most types of cancer than ever before. Wouldn't it be better to keep ourselves healthy in the first place?

Chiropractic can help our bodies work better. It's new, it's exciting, and, as I said before, it *works*. Millions have already discovered this. Today the majority of professional football, basketball, baseball, and hockey teams have chiropractors on call, whose job is to help million-dollar players perform at their peak.

Joe Montana is a good example. The former star quarterback who many think is the best who's ever played the game credits chiropractic with helping him play his best.

"The way I look at it is that it makes me feel better and I'm healthier and it keeps me on the field," said Montana, several years before he retired. "Chiropractic isn't just for a bad back or neck. It's about prevention so your body can function at optimum health. I don't see any reason why I shouldn't do it." Montana's entire family receives regular chiropractic spinal adjustments.

Celebrities such as Mel Gibson, Bruce Willis, Demi Moore, Raquel Welch, and Arnold Schwarzenegger are all enthusiastic chiropractic patients. So are Ronald Reagan and Newt Gingrich. From fitness experts like best-selling author Joyce Vedral to women's advocate Gloria Steinem, many well-known personalities rely on chiropractic to help keep them in top shape. You can, too. In the chapters ahead, you'll find exercises, nutrition advice, and mental techniques. Each is based on the chiropractic principle of unleashing the body's ability to function at one-hundred-percent effectiveness by eliminating what D. D. Palmer termed "pressure on nerves."

Although a trip to a chiropractor is necessary to make sure your nervous system is functioning at its best, the advice given in the pages ahead will get your nervous system functioning at a higher level than you've ever enjoyed, leading to fewer aches and pains, and a body with all the energy and vitality you need to live a healthy life.

I

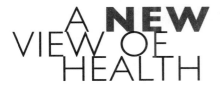

A NEW VIEW OF HEALTH

[health is an inside job]

I give a "Life Talk" for new patients every Wednesday night at my chiropractic office. The evening begins with the members of the group introducing themselves and sharing why they've become patients.

"Right shoulder pain," says a retired electrician whose golf game is suffering because of an aching arm.

"Dizziness and neck pain from an accident," says a young woman whose car was rear-ended while stopped at a traffic light.

"Back pain," notes a construction worker.

"Scoliosis," a teenager murmurs, using the medical term for curvature of the spine.

"Headaches," report several people in the group.

"Stress," sighs the owner of a small business, slumping in his chair after a long day at the office.

Most of us are bothered by similar health problems from time to time. But my Life Talks aren't about getting rid of these common symptoms. They're about going beyond relieving symptoms, toward experiencing total health.

I start my talks by asking, "What is health? What does health mean to you?" The group's answers are surprisingly consistent. Most say, "Health is feeling good." If you took a nationwide survey, I imagine the results would be about the same. Most people think that if you feel good, you're healthy.

Most people are wrong.

A CLEAN BILL OF HEALTH

Ironically, most health problems are caused by our belief that if we feel good, we're healthy. This is the reason why most middle-aged men and women carry aches and pains in their bodies the way suitcases carry clothing. It's why senior citizens spend their last years battling such degenerative diseases as arthritis, high blood pressure, and heart disease, and why so many die untimely deaths.

Feeling good can be deadly. For example, according to medical textbooks, it takes between seven and fifteen years before cancer cells in the breast grow to a lump you can feel during self examination. This means a woman could be doing self-exams for years, finding nothing, while in fact cancer is growing beneath her fingertips. She might feel great. But is she healthy?

Cancer often takes its victims by surprise, but what about something as common—and deadly—as a heart attack? Surely most people have early indications that there is trouble brewing. But in more than 50 percent of heart attack cases the first "symptom" is death. In other words, over half the time the person just drops dead.

We've all heard stories of a "healthy" middle-aged executive doing a common chore like mowing the lawn when suddenly a pain sears through his left arm. He drops to the ground. He feels as if an elephant were standing on his chest. Gasping for air, he dies of a massive heart attack.

Such commonplace stories shock us, slapping us in the face with a simple fact: a pain-free body isn't necessarily healthy. They also reveal the basic truth that although feeling good is often a benefit of health, it's not what health is.

So where did we get this idea that health is merely "feeling good"? The answer is as close as your medicine cabinet.

CAN'T BUY ME HEALTH

The United States has more medical doctors than any other country in the world. We have more hospitals, too. And more than half of the medical "breakthroughs" in treating disease take place right here.

Citing these statistics during our Wednesday-night talks, I ask my patients what they add up to. Many say, "A lot of money."

They're right. We're spending more than $800 billion a year on health care. What does all that money buy? One gem is fantastic emergency health care. If you're in a high-speed car accident, if your parachute doesn't open, or if you're otherwise burned, broken, or torn, there's no better place to be treated than in the United States.

Modern medicine is also great at replacing your body's original equipment. Kidney transplants and hip replacements are examples of "miracle" surgeries that greatly improve the quality of many people's lives.

Is there anything our expensive medical establishment *doesn't* buy? The World Health Organization (WHO) ranks countries for overall health. Where do we rank? When I ask patients at my Life Talks to guess, most give a high number. "First" is a popular answer.

That answer would be close—if this were 1932. In the early 1930s, the United States ranked second in overall health. Sadly, since then we've been dropping faster than a spoon through hot soup. Today we rank eighteenth, though 14 percent of our gross domestic product goes toward health care—a larger percentage than any other country in the world.

For all the money we spend, people in sixteen other nations enjoy a longer life span. Twenty other countries have a better infant survival rate.

How can we be swamped with doctors, hospitals, and high-tech medicine, and yet be getting less and less healthy?

When I first read these statistics, I called WHO and spoke with one of its public information officers.

"Surely these figures only apply to people who can't afford health care," I said. "For the majority of Americans this just can't be true." But, as I was told, recent statistics show that Americans as a group, even those with good health insurance, are getting less healthy. It's now estimated that one in four will develop heart disease. One in five will die of cancer.

The most appalling fact is that young people today are less healthy than at any time since the turn of the century.

Arnold Schwarzenegger, former chairman of the President's Council on Physical Fitness, reports the following statistics in his book, *Arnold's Fitness for Kids:*

- Recent studies on millions of American children aged five to seventeen revealed that 64 percent of them fail to meet minimum fitness standards.
- Obesity among children aged six through eleven is up by 54 percent since the 1960s, and super-obesity by as much as 98 percent, according to a 1987 study conducted by the Harvard School of Public Health.
- Fully 28 percent of children have high blood pressure. Nearly half have elevated levels of cholesterol. Almost 70 percent eat too much salt. Seventy-five percent have diets too rich in fats, and 67 percent show three or more risk factors for heart disease.

When we discuss these facts at our Wednesday-night talks, my patients will explain our predicament in a number of ways. Many say, "It's our lifestyle," or "We eat too much," or "We don't exercise enough," or "We're under too much stress."

These are all valid explanations. But there's something more basic. If you look at *why* we eat too much, fail to exercise, and are stressed out, you'll find the reason behind these unhealthy lifestyle choices.

THE MISINFORMATION AGE

I refuse to believe people don't want to be healthy. Why, then, do so many live in a way that creates aching bodies filled with disease? I believe that while there is a tremendous amount of wonderful information available on how to get healthy—get regular exercise, eat low-fat, low-salt food, don't smoke, and so on—we lack a basic understanding of what, exactly, is this thing called health.

When I ask new patients where they learn about health, most say, "From doctors." That's a nice thought. But when was the last time a doctor sat down with you for an hour to talk about getting healthier? According to recent statistics, the average time spent with a doctor during a typical office visit is eight minutes. Most people would find it difficult to prepare microwave popcorn in eight minutes, let alone learn how to take care of themselves.

We don't get most of our information about health from doctors. Like most information in the "communication age," we acquire it from the media, particularly television.

THE DRUG CONNECTION

According to CBS's "60 Minutes," pharmaceutical companies now spend more than $1 billion per month on advertising and promotion. That's more than is spent researching and developing their products. About one fifth of all television commercials advertise drugs. By the time the average child reaches eighteen years of age, he or she has seen twenty thousand hours of drug commercials.

All that marketing pays off. Americans now take more than half of all the drugs in the world, swallowing or injecting about 25 million doses each hour. There are more than 25,000 prescription potions and 200,000 over-the-counter drugs on the market, with the average American home containing twenty-nine different types.

Some Life Talk participants object when I point out these facts. They'll say, "Those commercials are selling products. They don't pretend to explain how to get healthier. It's not like they're trying to trick you." No, most aren't. But what do drug ads teach us?

My favorite drug commercial targets, as it says, "the person who needs a pain reliever several times a week." It begins by showing a pretty, smartly dressed young woman in her kitchen, cooking breakfast. The bottom of the television screen reads, "Monday Morning." It's the kind of day we'd all like to enjoy at the start of a week. Sunlight is pouring through a large picture window. You can almost hear the birds outside, chirping merrily. Suddenly the woman's son comes running through the kitchen. In his enthusiasm, he knocks over a pitcher of orange juice. In slow motion it falls, smashing on the floor. With glass flying everywhere, the woman is seized by a terrible headache. She grabs her head. The camera zooms in. Her head pulsates. Ba-boom! Ba-boom! Ba-boom! She takes some aspirin and, ahhh . . . the pain goes away.

The commercial continues, but now the bottom of the screen reads, "Wednesday Afternoon." The woman is bending over, lifting grocery bags out of her car trunk. Wham! Suddenly she's seized by a terrible backache. She grabs her flank. It pulsates. The camera zooms in. Ba-boom! Ba-boom! Ba-boom! Again she takes some aspirin, and the pain goes away.

This commercial's theme is repeated hundreds of times each day by other medicine makers. The message is always the same: As long as you can relieve the headache, backache, upset stomach, or vaginal yeast infection by taking a pill, syrup, or caplet, or by applying a cream, gel, or lotion, you're healthy again. In other words, if you develop symptoms that make you feel bad, you're unhealthy. The way to get healthy again is to get rid of the symptoms.

I've singled out drug advertisements for explaining this idea, but they're only the most obvious examples; our whole health system revolves around it. Let's go back to the doctor's office for our eight-minute visit. You tell the doctor what's bothering you. She gives you a prescription. If it doesn't work in a week, she gives you another. And so it continues. There may be some tests thrown in here and there. Surgery may cut out an offending organ. Finally, if all goes well, the symptoms fade away—at least temporarily.

THE FEELING TRAP

We're brought up to believe that maintaining health is a matter of eliminating pesky symptoms. *But symptoms aren't the problem.* Symptoms only point to an underlying problem. Unless the true cause is corrected, symptoms come back.

If "the person who needs a pain reliever several times a week" would stop and think, he or she might say, "If I need to keep taking these pills all the time, are they really fixing anything?" The packages for pain relievers say, "For the *temporary* relief of pain." (My italics.) The reason is that medications only mask pain while circulating in your blood. Once drugs get flushed from your body, the stage is set for more pain.

If we treated our cars the same way we do our heads when we take aspirin for a headache, it might go something like this: You're on vacation, driving your car to another state. Suddenly your temperature gauge starts blinking red. The light is a symptom brought on by an overheated engine.

Applying the same logic to your car as to your head, you might take an aspirin bottle out of your pocket and cover the flashing light! You've taken care of the symptom, but have you solved the problem?

WHEN SICK IS HEALTHY

Is there a healthier way to look at symptoms? During my Life Talks, I ask for symptoms associated with colds and flus. The list usually looks something like this:

- Sneezing and coughing
- Diarrhea and vomiting
- Fatigue
- Loss of appetite
- Pain
- Fever

Next I ask, "Why does your body sneeze and cough?" Everyone knows it's to get rid of germs. In fact, with each cough or sneeze, someone with a flu sprays hundreds of thousands of bacteria or viruses out of his or her body. Coughing also brings up mucus, produced as the body fights infection.

"Now, is it good or bad that your body expels the germs infecting it?" I ask. Everyone agrees it's good.

If you go to a Chinese restaurant and order chow mein, and along with it get ptomaine poisoning, is it good or bad that your body quickly dumps the poison through vomiting and diarrhea? What would happen if you ate the poison and *couldn't* get rid of it?

If you're fighting an infection, should you spend the day in aerobics classes or eating a five-course lunch? Do you think you'd get better faster if you rested and let the energy usually used to digest food be put to use fighting your infection?

How about pain? Say you're hammering nails while listening to the radio. A song takes you back to a pleasant memory. Your mind drifts and . . . pow! You miss the nail and slam your thumb. A terrible pain shoots up your arm. Good or bad? What would happen if your thumb couldn't produce pain and you kept daydreaming? Pain lets us know something is wrong.

The body has a reason for creating fevers, too: they act to speed up the action of our immune systems. A 1988 study traced two groups of children with measles. One group was left alone, and the other was given a medication to reduce fever. The group whose fevers were left to do their jobs recovered sooner.

Most people think that when they're sick and develop symptoms, they're unhealthy. But when you're sick, your body is actually working very hard, through sneezing, coughing, diarrhea, vomiting, pain, fatigue, and fever, to get you well. *All these symptoms are either warnings that something is wrong or signs of the body's attempts to heal itself.*

From watching drug commercials and observing our current medical system, you would never guess your body has the ability to heal itself. Chiropractors recognize your body's ability to heal. Instead of treating symptoms, they remove the interference that prevents your healing powers from getting you well and keeping you that way, thereby giving your body a chance to recuperate.

When I talk with people about these ideas, many say, "Oh, you're just against drugs because you're a chiropractor." I'm not against all drugs, all the time; sometimes they're necessary. If you wake up in the middle of the night with a pounding toothache, who am I to say you shouldn't take an aspirin until you can get to the dentist?

What I *am* opposed to is the idea that covering up or getting rid of symptoms allows us to gain full health, especially when talking about serious health problems.

For example, how about the person who is seventy pounds overweight, works at a high-stress job, doesn't exercise, and eats enough fat each day to grease a roller coaster? After a decade or two of living this lifestyle they (surprise!) develop symptoms of high blood pressure.

A majority of high-blood-pressure patients can cure themselves by eating a more nutritious diet, exercising regularly, and learning to relax, which together take about a half hour per day. Or they can bring the pressure down by taking medication. Which solution is best?

In our society, high blood pressure is often caused by a sedentary, high-stress lifestyle and a fat-rich diet, leading to hardening and narrowing of the arteries. As a person's arteries stiffen and shrink, his heart works harder to force blood out into the body, raising blood pressure. Does decreasing blood pressure with medications stop the arteries from shrinking and hardening? Not at all. In fact, with less pressure the clogging process can be speeded up.

Covering up the symptom of high blood pressure is only one example of how misinformation about health is killing us.

A NEW VIEW OF HEALTH

But if health isn't feeling good, what *is* it? Can we look at health in a different way, one that allows us to get healthier rather than only relieving our symptoms? I believe we can, and I think looking at the word *health* is a good place to start.

If you were back in elementary school and your teacher asked for the root word of "health," you'd probably say, "heal." And you'd be right; a big part of health is your body's ability to heal itself. We've seen how many symptoms reflect the body's attempts at self-healing. There are countless others.

For example, if you cut your finger and put a Band-Aid on it, does the Band-Aid heal the finger? Of course not, so there must be something *inside you* that knows how to heal the cut. The individual cells that are cut don't heal. They die. New cells are created to take their place. Most of what we call healing actually is the creation of new life. And while we know some of the mechanisms of healing, *why* those mechanisms go into action to create new cells out of peanut butter sandwiches and diet sodas will always be a mystery. But there is no mystery about one fact: without the ability to heal yourself, you wouldn't be alive to read this.

Health is also how well your body functions. In other words, a person whose liver, heart, spleen, lungs, gallbladder, and every other organ functions at 100 percent efficiency is much healthier than someone who has the same parts functioning at 60, 70, 80, or even 90 percent. So our new view of health must recognize that to get healthier we must allow our bodies to function better.

Health is not merely feeling good. Health is your body's ability to heal, and to function at a high level. The two are intimately connected, and strengthening that connection is what this book is all about.

Your liver performs more than two hundred functions at various times throughout the day. Can you name them all? How about fifty? Ten? At Life Talk, I write the numbers one through five on a presentation board and ask patients to list five liver functions. This gets a laugh, because no group can ever name five functions.

There's not a doctor in the United States who can sit down and write from memory all the functions of the liver and every other organ. But there's one "doctor" who can. This doctor knows every function of every cell in your body. Do you know where to find this doctor?

Inside you.

Doesn't it make sense that unless there was something inside you that controlled your liver, your liver couldn't work, because you're certainly not thinking about it all the time. If you get eight hours of sleep tonight, your heart will beat about thirty thousand times. If you had to think about making your heart beat, you wouldn't get much sleep.

Like your liver and heart, right now every other part of your body is functioning at a certain level. How? What's in control? When I ask patients which part of their body controls all the other parts, the answer is unanimous: the brain.

Let's see how the brain is wired to every part of you, allowing it to control and coordinate your body's every function. Let's learn about the most important part of you, your nervous system.

2

THE WORLD'S GREATEST DOCTOR LIVES INSIDE YOU

[how your nervous system keeps you healthy]

On page 18 is a picture of the greatest doctor in the world, your nervous system. Also shown are your skull and spine. They make up the two-story house where this personal-health guru lives.

The nervous system is made of three parts. Your *brain* sits in your skull, protected on all sides by hard bone. Your *spinal cord* is enclosed by your spine. It extends from your brain to your low back. *Nerves* branch off from the cord and blaze millions of trails into your body, not stopping until they end right beneath your skin.

Your nervous system keeps your body running. As you read this sentence, millions of **nerve impulses**—tiny electrical signals carrying information—are flashing back and forth over your nerves, as one part of your body communicates with others. Only a fraction as powerful as a telephone signal, these electrical flashes let you think, make your muscles work, and, through your senses, tell you about the world outside yourself.

TOP GUN

If you put every chiropractor, medical doctor, acupuncturist, physical therapist, and witch doctor in the world together in a laboratory, they wouldn't have a clue about how to grow a toenail. Yet your nervous system

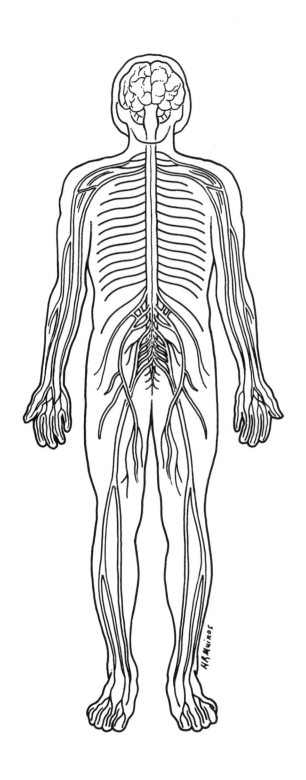

is growing ten of them right now. It's also keeping your heart beating, your lungs breathing, and your hands holding this book. How do the different parts of your nervous system work to keep you thriving?

Let's start at the top, with your brain, a creation that makes the latest, most powerful computer seem as technologically advanced as Tinker Toys.

It's said that if scientists tried to make a computer that could do all your brain does, it would be one hundred stories high and as wide as the state of Texas! This powerhouse is made of tiny cells. No one knows exactly how many brain cells are sitting between your ears, but estimates range from 10 billion to 100 billion.

The cells, known as *neurons,* look almost like bright stars. Branching off from their small centers are dozens of little roots, or *dendrites,* that reach out around the cell.

Nerve cells talk to each other with electricity. A tiny electrical impulse travels from the center, or *nucleus,* of one cell out over one of its dendrites. At the end of the dentrite there's a space about one millionth of an inch wide, called a *synapse.* The impulse jumps over this gap to a branch of the next cell.

"Every thought, every twitch of your finger, is an electrical event, or a series of electrical events," write Judith Hooper and Dick Teresi in their book on the brain, *The Three-Pound Universe.* "All the information that reaches you from the world—from the pattern of light and shadow that composes a face to the voice of the anchorman on the news—gets translated into a sequence of electrical pulses."

Your brain is always lit up with electrical patterns forming, shifting, and dissolving, because the electrical link between nerve cells forms and vanishes in an instant.

But your brain isn't just a three-pound bag of nerve cells that think they're spark plugs. Groups of cells get together and form different sections of your brain, each performing a different job. Together the parts of your brain form an incredibly powerful command post responsible for controlling and coordinating your body's every function.

Powerful as it is, without a way to speak with the rest of you, your brain would be a frustrated genius locked in a dark closet. That's why you have a spinal cord.

YOU'VE GOT A LOT OF NERVES

Your spinal cord is a thick bundle of nerves. It exits from your skull and cascades down inside your spine, ending up three to five inches above your waist.

Many people associate the spinal cord with traumatic accidents—rightly so, because when the spinal cord is injured, it often results in loss of the use of arms and/or legs.

For example, every few years a professional or college football player takes a severe blow to the head and neck and ends up in a wheelchair. A fractured neck bone has cut into his spinal cord, disconnecting the player's brain from his muscles.

Executioners use the vulnerability of the cord when they hang prisoners. As the unfortunate felon drops from the gallows and literally hits the end of his rope, the force breaks the second bone of the neck, which promptly slices through the cord, causing nearly instantaneous death.

The vital messages traveling through your spinal cord would be useless if they didn't have a way to get out into your body. That is the job of your nerves.

LONG-DISTANCE DIRECT

Your nerves are your body's telephone wires. As they exit the cord, they're packed into big bundles, like electrical cables. Then, almost immediately, they start branching out. As they travel farther from the spine, they split into ever-smaller threads, weaving their way through every inch of you. They are so numerous that if every part of you but your nerves disappeared, your friends could still recognize you, because your nerves would form a 3-D image of incredible detail.

Though your nerves are like telephone wires, your body's nervous system is much more complex than any telephone network. Even if there were a thousand times more people in the United States and each had a portable cellular phone, the telephone system still wouldn't be as intricately connected as the nerves in your body.

For example, for you to turn this page, your brain will have to send out hundreds of thousands of nerve impulses. These bits of electricity will shoot out of your brain to muscles in your shoulders, arms, hands, and fingers.

Will you need to think about contracting your shoulder's deltoid muscle or your fingers' interosseus muscles? Thankfully not. Just think of turning the page, and presto!—signals to all the appropriate muscles are dispatched.

Your brain's control over your glands and other organs is no less dramatic than its coordination of your muscles.

Your glands are organs that produce hormones, or chemical messengers. Like nerve impulses, hormones communicate information from one part of your body to another. For example, in pregnant women the brain signals a gland to produce a hormone called *relaxin*. This hormone travels throughout the bloodstream and relaxes ligaments in the expecting mother. Without relaxin to loosen the ligaments of her birth canal, it would be nearly impossible for a mother to push a baby into the world.

Like glands, all the organs in your body are controlled by your brain through nerves. For example, as you read this, your spleen is sorting through your red blood cells and recycling the ones that are worn out. Your brain controls your spleen's function so you can pay attention to more important things, such as what's for dinner.

SENSE-ATIONAL

Some of the most important nerve connections in your body are the ones between your brain and your eyes, ears, skin, tongue, and nose. These sense organs use receptor cells to give your brain information about what's happening in the world around you. Receptor cells can turn sensations as varied as the warmth of the sun and the smell of bubbling tomato sauce into electrical impulses that travel along nerves to your brain, where they're used to make order out of this sometimes crazy world.

Your brain changes your body with each bit of sensory information it receives. When it's hot you sweat, when it's cold you shiver, when you smell honey you think of—whatever you think of, for your brain is filled with personal experiences gathered through your senses over the years.

Many techniques in this book use the connections between your senses and your brain to make your nervous system work better. Let's see how your senses influence the way your nervous system works.

TOUCH ME, FEEL ME

When you touch something, receptors in your skin transform that experience into electrical impulses that race to your brain, telling it about the object's shape and texture. But the sense of touch doesn't stop there; different skin receptors also allow you to feel pressure, heat, cold, movement, vibration, and pain.

In addition, millions of receptors embedded in muscles throughout your body feed information to your brain, telling it about how your muscles are working. This lets your brain know where your arms and legs are, and if they are tense or relaxed. Without these receptors, it would be impossible to close your eyes and touch your finger to your nose.

If you've ever received a soothing massage, you've learned how touch affects your nervous system. Receptors in your skin pick up sensations of warmth and delight from another person's caring touch. At the same time, muscle receptors note a release of tension. Your brain interprets these signals as signs that everything is right with the world, and you feel relaxed.

NOW HEAR THIS

When a drummer plays, his drum shakes and makes the air around it vibrate, creating sound waves. Your ear transforms those waves into nerve signals and sends them to your brain, where you "hear" the drum.

Sounds from the outside world affect our emotions and thoughts. A jackhammer's rat-a-tat-tat on a crowded city street can make us feel physically attacked, while top-ten pop music can have us bouncing in our seat. Today, sound researchers are pushing our knowledge of the sound/mind connection even further, developing soundtracks that can enhance relaxation, creativity, memory, and learning.

A CLEAR VIEW

Of all your senses, your eyes are the most important. Research indicates that four-fifths of what you remember is something you've seen.

Receptors in your eyes change light into electrical impulses, which your brain translates into pictures. You actually "see" in your brain.

Like all sensory information, visual images are fed to the part of your brain that creates emotions. Soothing images, such as a gentle sunset, calm us. The violent murders filmed with gut-wrenching realism in action/adventure movies jangle every cell in our bodies.

TASTE OF THE TOWN

Your tongue is almost solid muscle. But tiny taste buds covering its surface sense flavors, send this information to your brain, and this can affect how your brain works.

As we'll learn, putting a chocolate bar in your mouth automatically impacts how your nervous system works.

A NOSE FOR NEWS

A million years ago, we relied on our noses to pick the scent of an animal from the wind. Today our noses remain as sensitive as wallflowers at a high school dance.

Smells are how we interpret chemicals inhaled through the nose. Nerve receptors "read" the chemicals, changing this information into electrical impulses.

Smells profoundly affect how our nervous systems work, especially our memory and emotions. That's why smelling oregano can remind you of your favorite Italian restaurant. Today the link between "scent power" and nervous system function is being rediscovered. Aromatherapy—the use of scents to influence the nervous system—is a fast-growing field. As we'll see, just inhaling lavender can calm us, while a smell such as tangerine can revitalize us from the inside out.

CONTROL FREAK

With your brain connected to your body through nerves, you're equipped with a marvelous communication system. The nerves let your brain tell your big toe what to do. And if your big toe happens to hit the bedpost in the middle of the night, it can very quickly tell your brain that it's unhappy.

Of course, there are many mysteries surrounding why and how the brain works. Why does your brain make your skin blush when you recall the time in sixth grade when the teacher embarrassed you in front of the class? Nobody knows. Most likely, nobody will ever know, though a lot of people are trying to figure it out.

What we *do* know is that many of the signals that control and coordinate your body are triggered in response to incoming information from your senses. Your brain changes your body in response to what you experience.

For example, let's say Mark gets a new job as a ditch digger. His boss gives him a brand-new shovel and says, "Go to it." Mark starts digging ditches eight hours a day.

At the end of a month, what will have happened to Mark's hands? Chances are they would be stronger and callused. What will have happened to the shovel? It will have become dull and worn.

Unless the stresses we face are overwhelming, our bodies get stronger with use, because we have nervous systems. So if you start digging ditches, your body sends signals to your brain, saying, "Hey! We're under a lot of stress down here! Do something!" Your nervous system then adapts you to this new stress by strengthening your hands and arms.

Another amazing feature of this mind-body link is that *your brain can change your body in response to thoughts alone.*

Let's say you're a winning contestant on a television game show. Your prize is that you've been given five minutes to run through a grocery store, filling shopping carts with food and prizes.

You're standing at the front of the store, television lights glaring in your eyes, hands gripping your cart. What will your heart be doing? Even though you're standing still, it will be trying to pound its way out of your chest. Blood will be surging through you like water through a fire hose. Your eyes will be extremely sensitive. Colors will be brighter. Packages on the shelves will show up in greater contrast. You'll breathe twice as fast.

All this will be happening *in anticipation* of your upcoming treasure hunt, even though you're standing still, telling the game-show host about your family and hometown.

Your nervous system's wonderful control and coordination capabilities don't always lead to well-being, however. For example, one of the most hotly researched areas in health today is how negative thoughts and emotions can adversely affect one's health and well-being.

THE SAFETY PIN CYCLE

About the easiest way to think about how nerves connect your brain and body is to imagine a safety pin. The pin has a top and bottom and is connected by a loop of wire. Your brain-body connection works the same way, with nerves flowing out from your brain into your body, and other nerves flowing from your body up to your brain. *When nerve impulses flow unobstructed around this loop, good health naturally flourishes, because the brain is controlling and coordinating your health with 100 percent efficiency.*

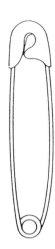

INTELLIGENT LIFE IN YOUR UNIVERSE

To say that nerve impulses are just tiny bits of electricity is like saying sunshine is just a bit of the sun cast into space. Sunlight carries energy and is the key to life on the surface of the earth. Nerve impulses carry intelligence in the form of information that keeps your body running.

It's the intelligence carried in nerve impulses that creates health inside you. That intelligence knows how to make a baby, turn a thought into a broken heart, and heal a cut finger without a bandage. If you want to build health, you need to keep that intelligence flowing.

I realized this one summer. My only brother had just died. At the time I was driving quite a distance to work every day, which gave me time to think. As so often happens when a loved one dies, I was brimming with an appreciation for life in all its forms.

This was particularly true of nature. A nice sunset could bring me to tears. I used to imagine that Robert's spirit was contained in shafts of sunlight, in billowy clouds, in gusts of wind. It was in this state that I wrote the following, titled "As Flowers Bloom":

> *Can the key to health be found in a tiger lily? This summer I realized it can.*
>
> *Beginning in May, I began traveling to work on long stretches of country road. As the sun shone through stands of green pines, I'd drive along asphalt trails forgotten by road maps. As I drove, I noticed bunches of*

bright wildflowers growing along the road: tiny hot-air balloons that Mother Nature had tethered to earth.

After a few weeks I had my favorite patches of tiger lilies and wild roses. I'd pull over, stop, and, using scissors from my briefcase, snip a few blossoms. I'd carry these into my chiropractic office, where I'd begin my day by arranging a bouquet in a vase on the reception desk.

Then, one Monday, I noticed that my patches of tiger lilies had been joined, seemingly overnight, by huge fields of brown-eyed Susans. Small meadows of these cheerful flowers lined the road, as if a floral carpet had been laid out over the weekend.

This precisely timed flourishing of flowers struck me as nature's wisdom at its simplest and most profound. No frantic florist, working under a strict deadline, rushes around telling flowers when to bloom. But they know.

They know exactly what week, out of the fifty-two weeks that make up our calendars, to throw open their brilliant shutters and let the sun wash over them. Not only that, but this timing is affected by everything natural. Rainfall, sunlight, temperature, and probably dozens of other influences we can't imagine all go into a flower's decision to blossom.

Thinking about this, I was struck by nature's intelligence. For it can't be anything less than an all-knowing interconnectedness that allows nature to be so beautifully orchestrated.

Wouldn't it be wonderful to tap into that intelligence? To let the same force that can paint country roads a hundred colors bring our bodies to full bloom?

Well, we can. That same intelligence of nature runs freely through our bodies. Just as nature knows exactly when tiger lilies should burst open and trumpet their orange symphonies, it knows what your body needs to stay healthy.

Flowers are the bows nature uses to gift-wrap herself. We gather them in bunches and marvel at the incomprehensible genius that shapes such beauty. Yet we are shaped by this same genius, and nature flows through us as surely as through a rose.

The founders of chiropractic realized that one of the keys to health was the correct flow of intelligence through the body's nerves. They labeled the information carried by the nerves "innate intelligence," calling it an "inborn intelligence responsible for maintaining all living things in existence."

They developed chiropractic to keep this intelligence flowing through the body, and summed up their thoughts in such maxims as "The power that made the body heals the body."

B. J. Palmer, the son of chiropractic's founder, D. D. Palmer, put it this way:

> *Chiropractic teaches that the life principle, or Innate Intelligence, intelligently selects and assembles chemical elements found in human anatomy; it builds organs of the body for certain purposes, and then controls and governs their function and activities by means of these mental impulses created in the brain and sent over nerves to every tissue cell in the body.*
>
> *It is obvious that impairment of the brain or nerve tissue will interfere with the normal creation, transmission and expression of mental impulses, with the result that the cells which these nerves supply will not receive or express the proper command; will not coordinate or work in harmony with the rest of the organism, and then we have a condition of dis-ease, or lack of ease.*

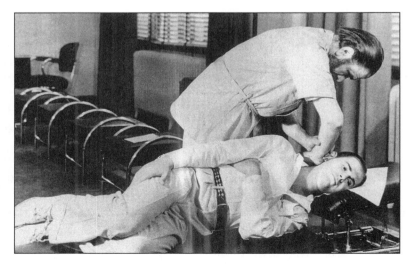

B. J. Palmer giving a chiropractic adjustment at his research clinic.

HOUSING CRISIS

In studying the nervous system, B. J. Palmer and other chiropractors at the beginning of the twentieth century asked, "How can this wonderful system we're equipped with, whereby the brain controls the body using nerves, develop problems?"

They found the answer in your spine, the house where the greatest doctor in the world lives. Let's look at how that house is built.

In your body the brain sits on top of your spine, protected by hard bone, your skull.

Like the skull, the spine protects the spinal cord with a shell of hard bone. Instead of being solid, however, the spine is made up of twenty-four bones, called *vertebrae*, stacked on top of one another like building blocks. Holes near the back of the bones create a tunnel for the spinal cord. Sandwiched between the bones, looking like squashed water balloons, are "disks." Tough yet flexible, they help us twist and bend, and act as shock absorbers.

If you move your hand to the back of your neck and press in, you can feel little bumps underneath the skin. What you're feeling are the tips of your seven neck bones (cervical vertebrae).

Usually you can feel a large bump right at the base of your neck. In most people, this is the seventh bone in the neck, or the first of twelve mid-back bones (thoracic vertebrae). Your mid-back bones differ from others in the spine because they have ribs attached to them.

The bottom of your spine is made up of five large low-back bones (lumbar vertebrae). Using your thumbs, find the spot right above your waist where there's a scooped-out area. If you push in, you can feel the bones of your low back.

Below the low back sits the wide, thick tailbone, or sacrum. Shaped like an upside-down triangle, it forms a foundation on which the rest of your spine sits.

Your spine must be stable enough to support your upper body, but flexible enough to let you move. Strong support and easy flexibility usually go together about as well as ballerinas and barbells. But your spine ingeniously blends the two opposite functions.

For example, the front half of a spinal bone is wide and thick. Shaped

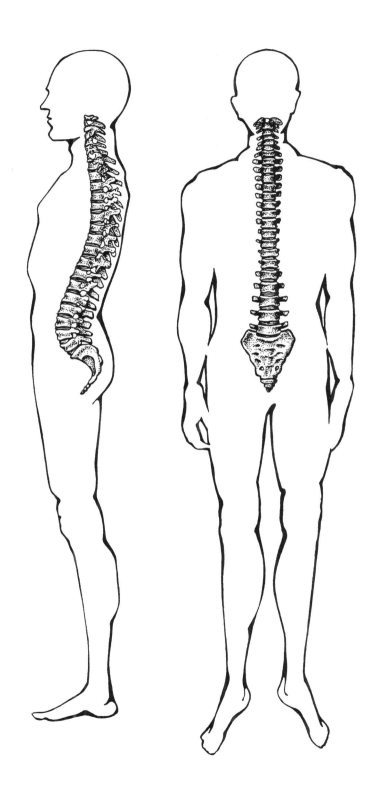

like a tree stump, this part carries a lot of weight. The back of the bone (the part you can feel under your skin) is shaped very differently. Sticking out like a—well, like a spine—the back is thin and narrow, with smooth, flat areas that come together with other bones to form joints.

To get an idea of how spinal joints work, put your hands together in a praying position and rub. The joints in your back move in a similar way, sliding smoothly on one another. If bones become misaligned, their smooth action can become jammed, causing problems.

PROBLEMS IN PARADISE

To sum up, in order to stay healthy, you need a nervous system functioning at 100 percent, so it can control and coordinate your body.

What happens when the greatest doctor in the world loses her or his control/coordination abilities? Let's see what happens when your inner doctor is overloaded.

3

THE WORLD'S GREATEST DOCTOR IS OVERLOADED

[how nervous system overload creates dis-ease]

The telephone call would change my life forever. I was in my first week of residency at chiropractic college, answering phones in the school's public clinic.

The woman caller introduced herself as Susan. She'd heard of the college's clinic from a neighbor. Her friend had suffered from headaches for many years until coming to the clinic, where they vanished under chiropractic care.

"My little girl is twelve years old. She hasn't been to school in two weeks. She's vomiting, she can't sleep, she can't eat anything without throwing up, and she says her head is killing her," Susan reported. Her daughter, Jodi, was scheduled in two days to see a neurologist, a medical doctor specializing in nerve disorders. Susan wanted to see if something could be done right away.

"Can you recommend a resident who's really good?" she asked.

"I'd be happy to help your little girl," I said with nervous excitement.

"Are you good?" asked Susan.

"Yes, I am," I said, hoping I was right.

I made the appointment for an hour later, hung up the phone, and felt sick to my stomach. I was worried. Twelve-year-olds don't get severe headaches. The textbooks I'd studied said that migraine headaches, vomiting, sleeplessness, and loss of appetite in a girl that age could mean only one thing: a brain tumor. Even if it wasn't a tumor, I wasn't convinced that chiropractic would work when delivered by my inexperienced hands.

My clinic director was also worried about a tumor. He and I examined Jodi for two hours before he gave the go-ahead to take X rays of her neck and treat her.

The X rays showed that the first bone in Jodi's neck had shifted dramatically to the left. I believed that was the source of her headaches. The nerves coming out of the spine at that level travel to the head. The intelligence that keeps the body working correctly uses these nerves to control the muscles and blood vessels on the scalp. When the first bone shifts out of position, it can "pinch" these nerves, causing a loss of control by the nervous system, producing headaches.

By the time we got Jodi into a treatment room, she'd been at the clinic for three hours. The room was small and bare. It contained a single treatment table, a small desk, and a chair.

The table was designed to help chiropractors move bones in a patient's neck. It had a special piece at one end, shaped like a flat box. I told Jodi to lie down on her side so that her head rested on this headpiece.

Using a small lever, I "popped" the headpiece up, so that Jodi's head was raised about two inches. With enough pressure, the headpiece was designed to give way, so that it dropped—along with the patient's head—to its starting position.

I placed my left hand just underneath Jodi's left ear, on the first bone in her neck. I took a deep breath, exhaled slowly, and then snapped my arms down and back, creating a thrust that shot into Jodi's neck and dropped her head with a loud thump.

I stepped back and turned to Susan. Her mouth was hanging open. She stared at me as though I had just thrown Jodi out a window.

I reached down and gently sat Jodi up on the table. "Are you okay?" I asked.

There was no need to worry, but I wanted to assure Susan that her daughter had survived my tender mercies. While the description of this neck adjustment might sound dangerous, it actually involves very little force. In school we practiced the adjustment using raw eggs. The egg was placed on the chiropractic table's headpiece, simulating a patient's neck. You had to thrust fast enough to make the table's headpiece drop without breaking the egg. When you experience this adjustment as a patient, you feel a quick tap from your chiropractor's hand and your head dropping down two inches, where it comes to an abrupt but well-cushioned stop.

Jodi said she felt fine as I lifted her up.

"All right, let's see how that works," I said.

"Is that all you're going to do?" asked Susan, who, after sitting through three hours of examinations, had just witnessed a "treatment" that took a tenth of a second.

"That's all she needs," I said.

I couldn't sleep that night, I was so excited. The next morning I called Susan.

"How's Jodi doing?" I asked.

"Leonard, I don't know how to thank you," she said. "Jodi's father and I couldn't believe it. Last night she came home and went right to sleep. This morning she got up without a headache, ate breakfast, and went to school. She's feeling fine."

I never again doubted the power of chiropractic—even when delivered through my hands—to get sick people well.

Two years after I graduated from chiropractic college, a woman and her three-year-old daughter who had been in an auto accident were sitting in my office, telling me about the wreck. The little girl, Valera, had large, deep, open sores on her face. I asked her mother if Valera had been cut with flying glass during the accident.

"Oh no, she's had those sores on her face since she was eight months old," said the mother. "The doctors say she's allergic to bread."

I was puzzled, not only because most eight-month-olds don't eat bread, but because, if that was the case, why would she still be eating it and causing such ghastly-looking sores?

"I really didn't understand the doctor," said Valera's mother upon further questioning. "She doesn't eat bread now, but those sores just stay there."

Two weeks after starting chiropractic care, Valera's skin was as smooth as silk. It was as if someone had taken an eraser to her sores, smoothing them away to expose the beautiful skin underneath. The nerves carrying information to the skin on her face had been restored to proper working order. As her skin began receiving the right information from her brain, Valera's skin healed.

Just yesterday in my office, I received some great news. For the past few years, Jacob, an eight-year-old boy, had wet his bed almost every night. He reported yesterday that he'd been dry every night since his first visit to our office four days ago. His mother, who'd spent thousands of dollars on various treatments, couldn't believe a chiropractor could get such tremendous results when everything else had failed.

During the past two years I've kept track of our success with bedwetting patients. Out of the eight children brought to our clinic for this problem, five completely stopped their bedwetting under chiropractic care, and two significantly improved. Usually these children have fallen and knocked their tailbones out of alignment. The misaligned tailbone then puts pressure on the nerves controlling urinary function. When the nerve pressure is relieved, the bedwetting stops.

The very next patient I saw after Jacob was a man in his sixties, who originally came to our clinic because of back pain. After listening to Jacob tell me about his progress, the man said, "Doc, I wasn't going to say anything about this, but before starting here last week, I'd thought about buying adult diapers because I was leaking in my underwear all the time. Since I started coming here, I haven't had that problem." He laughed as he told me that his co-workers had started calling him "Speedy" because of how much better he was walking.

Such results are extremely gratifying. In the past month, two patients in our office have reported that their eyesight has improved since they've become chiropractic patients! Again, when nerve pressure is relieved, the body can use the increased nerve flow to establish a higher state of health, which often shows up in surprising ways.

The above examples demonstrate what can happen when a person whose nervous system has lost its ability to control and coordinate health has this power restored.

TRUE LIES

When I tell people about some of the results my patients achieve under chiropractic care, they don't believe me. At dinner one night I told my mother-in-law about a little girl who had been brought to me because her neck was hurting, and after a week of care her chronic asthma disappeared. My mother-in-law expressed doubt. "That's just not possible! You think you can cure anything!" I explained that I never try to cure individuals of their symptoms; I leave that job to the body of the person I'm working on. I wasn't even aware of this girl's asthma problem before her mother told me about it.

Frankly, if I weren't a chiropractor and hadn't witnessed such cases, I might doubt these stories myself. And yet they are common occurrences, happening every day in chiropractic offices around the world. Every chiropractor I know experiences these kinds of "miracle" cases.

Why? How can one person be relieved of headaches, another of bedwetting, a third made to see better, and a fourth have her skin clear up because a chiropractor has improved the functioning of their nervous systems?

The answer is that chiropractors don't treat heads, bladders, eyes, or skin. By relieving nerve pressure, they release the ability of their patients' bodies to heal all these ailments and many more. They set free the intelligence carried in the nerve impulses flowing from the brain to the body and from the body up to the brain. When they do this, the body heals itself.

BLOCK PARTY

What happens to create nerve pressure in the first place?

Most nerve pressure is caused by "blocks"—areas in our bodies where nerve impulses become trapped or distorted. Blocks develop when our nervous systems become overloaded owing to physical, emotional, mental, or chemical stress.

Blocks formed when your nervous system is overwhelmed by physical stress are the easiest to understand.

For example, recently a construction worker named Doug came into my clinic with tears streaming down his agonized face. He was limping, hanging on to his wife and son for support. Doug had been on a ladder, working on a house, when several roof trusses—large wooden A-frame structures weighing hundreds of pounds—fell off the roof and onto his back, knocking him to the ground. His neck was as stiff as a pipe when I examined it. He couldn't move an inch without wincing from pain. X rays revealed two broken bones in his mid-back, with many more twisted out of their normal position.

When confronted with the tremendous force thrust upon it, Doug's nervous system had been overloaded. As bones broke, his nervous system responded to this stress by immediately sending signals to the muscles in his back. The muscles locked into spasm, creating a vise, preventing further injury.

Several bones had been twisted out of their normal position by the impact. Now spasms wrenched these and other bones in the area farther out of alignment, causing them to "pinch" nerves in the surrounding area. Doug's nervous system confronted an overwhelming stress by adapting as best it could.

However, as William Hanna points out in his excellent book *Somatics*, which explores how our nervous systems adapt our bodies to stress, these overload episodes leave a legacy:

> *The brain is an adaptive organ. It responds to the events of our lives in whatever way is necessary in order to survive and keep going. But, because the brain directly or indirectly controls all our bodily functions, this means that our entire body reflects what has happened to us during our lifetimes.*

As Hanna points out, overload creates a blocked area of the body that, without care, forever loses the ability to function at 100 percent efficiency.

In Doug's case, we sent him to the emergency room. After he'd had several days of bed rest, we began moving back into position the bones knocked out of alignment during his accident. Meanwhile, his body began healing his fractures. He also was put on an exercise program that included swimming, stretching, and strengthening exercises.

If Doug's spine hadn't received treatment after his accident, it would have developed permanent problems. For the rest of his life, bones in his back would have been locked into an abnormal position, pinching nerves.

The muscles in his back would never again have worked as before. His back would constantly have sent signals to his brain saying, "Hey! I'm in trouble!" and his brain would have continued to create spasmed muscles as a way to protect Doug from further injury.

As in Doug's case, nervous system overload usually results in two types of blocks, either of which can create nerve pressure. One occurs when your muscles spasm, affecting nerve function, the other when joints become misaligned and start pinching nerves, again affecting function.

Muscle spasms and joint misalignments usually go hand in hand. Tight muscles often pull bones out of alignment, and misalignments cause muscles to tighten in an effort to realign the bones. Both create trouble by blocking or distorting the normal flow of nervous system energy in our bodies.

In short, overload creates **blocks,** leading to **dis-ease,** which produces symptoms.

ENTRY-LEVEL CONDITIONS

Before we look at the emotional, mental, and chemical causes of nervous system overload, we can't overlook one of the most common causes of physical overload to our nervous system: the birth process. At birth, many children's necks are twisted and pulled, pinching nerves in the area.

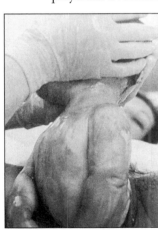

Twist and shout. The birth process sometimes causes pinched nerves in the neck.

Miranda was a little two-month-old who was driving her parents crazy with colic, a condition in which babies develop uncontrollable fits of crying. Miranda's mother told me that owing to complications, the doctor who delivered the baby used forceps, metal tongs used to grab a baby's head and pull it from the birth canal.

Upon feeling Miranda's neck I could guess what had happened: Her first and second cervical vertebrae had been shifted out of position at birth, pinching on nerves, causing pain and irritability. With my fingertips, I contacted the first and second bones in the child's neck. Babies are incredibly easy to work on because the pressure required to move their bones is minimal. Using about as much force as it would take to dent a loaf of bread, I moved the bones back. That night the colic stopped.

Many misalignments brought on by the birth process fix themselves. Sometimes, however, the results of this physical form of nervous system overload remain, with children developing colic, chronic ear infections, respiratory problems, and frequent colds; later in life they may experience headaches and neck pain.

IT'S ALL IN YOUR MIND

Think about the last time you were really angry. Do you remember how tight the muscles in your jaw, neck, and shoulders felt? Other emotions work the same way. Each produces a matching set of muscular reflexes in your body.

William Hanna explains the phenomenon this way:

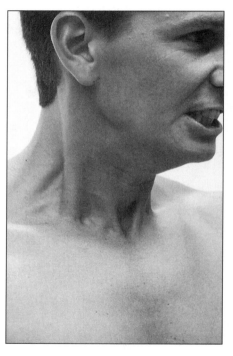

In a clench. Strong emotions cause muscles to tighten throughout our bodies.

> *The fact is that, during the course of our lives, our sensory-motor systems continually respond to daily stresses and traumas with specific muscular reflexes. These reflexes, repeatedly triggered, create habitual muscular contractions, which we cannot—voluntarily—relax. . . . [B]ecause this occurs in the central nervous system, we are not aware of it, yet it affects us to our very core.*

Mental stress affects our bodies just as much as emotional tension. My sister-in-law used to work in our clinic's insurance department. You could always tell when she was having a stressful day, because her shoulders would be raised up close to her earlobes.

"Hey, Trice," I'd say, "did you leave your neck at home today?" When she realized how she was holding her shoulders, she'd thank me, take a deep breath, and let her shoulders sink back to their normal level.

Most of the time our muscles relax when we let go of emotional or mental tension. However, if we always feel anxious our muscles become tense and tight all the time.

Hanna explains how this happens through what he calls *habituation:*

> *Habituation is the simplest form of learning. . . . When the same bodily response occurs over and over again, its pattern is gradually "learned" at an unconscious level. Habituation is a slow, relentless adaptive act, which ingrains itself into the functional patterns of the central nervous system. When you see someone with a stooped posture, you're looking at a posture that has been imprinted in the neuromuscular system by habituation. Anxiety accumulates in our lives, layer upon layer, creating ever rising levels of habitual muscular tension in our jaws, eyes, brows, necks, shoulders, arms, chests, bellies and legs.*

If we keep tightening our muscles in response to emotional and mental stress, soon our body develops problems. Tight muscles can tug bones out of position, putting pressure on nerves. Such muscles can also restrict blood flow. Pain can develop, with the brain responding by tightening the area further.

THE CHEMISTRY OF STRIFE

Just as serious, though less understood than the physical, emotional, and mental causes of nervous system overload, is overload brought on by chemical stress. D. D. Palmer recognized the significance of chemical stress early on in his development of chiropractic, writing:

> *The poison, acting on certain nerves, irritates their structure. They in turn contract muscles which draw vertebrae out of alignment, thereby impinging upon nerves which go and affect certain portions of the body.*

Studies have since shown that food additives, tobacco smoke, air pollution, drugs, and many other chemical substances can cause a loss of nerve flow within the body.

IN A PINCH

We've seen how nerves are like telephone wires. What happens to a telephone wire when a tree falls on it? Do you think the line might develop some static? That's what happens when bones start pinching the nerves coming out of your spine. Vital messages coming down from the brain become distorted, and the body begins working at less than 100 percent efficiency.

An easy way to think about this is to imagine water flowing through a hose. Say you're using a garden hose to water flowers, and someone comes up behind you and steps on the hose. What happens to the flow of water? If the pressure on the hose isn't released, won't the flowers start to wither?

Chiropractors have a special name for misaligned bones that pinch nerves: **subluxations.** My definition of a subluxation is "a minor misalignment of the spine causing nerve interference." I like to say "minor misalignment" because many times only a slight movement of the bone from where it's supposed to be causes the nerves around it to function less effectively.

In your body, when nerves are pinched by subluxations the organs and muscles at the end of those nerves begin working at less than 100 percent. Studies show that even a small pressure on spinal nerves causes a drastic decrease in their ability to work.

For example, in 1988, at the University of Colorado, a researcher focusing on how the spine works devised the following gruesome experiment: Instead of charging the usual $25,000, he gave cats free back surgeries in which their spines were exposed.

The nerves exiting the spine were hooked to instruments measuring their function. Weights were then placed on the nerves to see how much function was lost. With the weight of a dime on it, a spinal nerve lost up to 60 percent of its normal nerve flow. What effect do you think that would have on the organs that nerve was sending signals to? (I don't approve of this type of experimentation, but the evidence it provided helped establish the scientific validity of chiropractic care.)

Other studies have demonstrated what happens to the human body when subluxations decrease nerve supply. Dr. Henry Winsor, a medical doctor, was inspired by chiropractic literature to experiment and see if there was a relationship between subluxations and organ disease. In a series of three studies done at the University of Pennsylvania in the 1920s, he dissected seventy-five human and twenty-two cat cadavers. Of 221 organs found to be diseased, 212 were supplied by nerves that were being pinched by spinal subluxations. For example, all twenty-six cadavers showing lung disease had subluxations in the upper back, where the nerves sending messages to the lungs exit the spine. The field of somato-visceral disease (the study of how the body's structure affects organ function) is booming today, proving what chiropractors have been saying for a hundred years.

THE PAIN GAME

Although loss of function is the most dangerous result of subluxations and other blocks in our bodies, pain is what alerts most of us to their presence. As nerves are pinched, they often shoot off pain signals like fireworks on the Fourth of July.

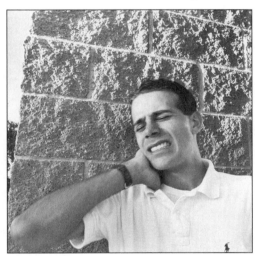

For example, one morning last week, Constance came into my clinic complaining of "terrible" neck pain. She'd been on vacation the week before, sleeping in an uncomfortable bed; the previous day's drive home had been long.

When she awoke in the morning, she couldn't move her neck. Sharp, shooting pain grabbed her with any movement. The medical

Pressure gauge. Neck pain often results from pinched nerves.

term for this common condition is *torticollis*. It's caused when neck bones—usually the second or fifth cervical vertebra—become misaligned and pinch nerves, which then cause pain and muscle spasms in the neck. We removed the subluxations in Constance's neck, and by afternoon she was turning her head again without pain.

Protecting Your Nerves

Your spine is uniquely designed to protect your **spinal cord** (the main carrier of messages to and from your brain) and **spinal nerves** (the "secondary carriers" of messages from your spinal cord to the rest of your body).

Vertebrae are spinal bones with openings to house and protect both your spinal cord and the nerve roots that branch to the rest of your body.

Your **spinal cord** runs from your brain down the middle of your spine through openings in your vertebrae.

Facets are joints between vertebrae that glide smoothly as you move your spine.

Nerves branch from your spinal cord and travel from openings between your vertebrae to the rest of your body.

Muscles support your spine and help it move.

Ligaments are strong, cable-like tissues that connect your vertebrae together.

Disks are "shock absorbers" and "spacers" between your vertebrae. They protect the vertebrae, spinal cord, and nerves.

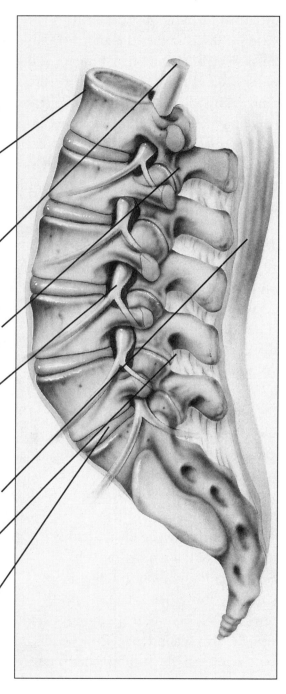

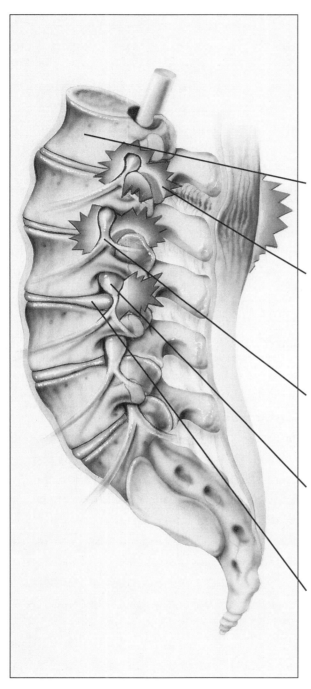

Subluxation: A Cause of Spinal Problems

Because the many parts of your spine work so closely together, a subluxation may cause problems in your vertebrae, nerves, facets, muscles, ligaments, disks, or blood vessels.

Misaligned vertebrae may irritate your nerves and cause your ligaments and muscles to stretch unevenly.

Sprained ligaments and **strained muscles** do not provide adequate support for the vertebrae, and can restrict or increase the normal movement of vertebral joints.

"Locked" facets may irritate the nerves and ligaments surrounding them, causing back and neck pain.

Irritated or **"pinched" nerves** may cause pain, numbness, or other problems in your spine or in other parts of your body.

Bulging or **ruptured disks** may place pressure against the nerve roots or spinal cord and may cause pain or numbness in your neck, back, arm, or leg.

AS TIME GOES BY

While pain lets most people know they have pinched nerves, many patients walking into a chiropractor's office are bringing in subluxations they've had for five, ten, fifteen, or even twenty years. All that time their bodies may have been pain-free, even while working at less than 100 percent.

Claire had worked as a typist for seventeen years when she came to see me because of carpal tunnel syndrome, a condition in which the hands, wrists, and forearms can become extremely painful.

The first thing Claire noticed was that her wrists and fingers began hurting. Within three months she began experiencing numbness in her hands. Soon this became mixed with sharp, shooting pains stinging up into her forearms. The pain often woke her from sleep during the night. Like many carpal tunnel sufferers, she described the pain "as if someone were sticking me with knives."

Interestingly, the lower part of Claire's neck had been misaligned years before in a car accident. The accident created spasmed muscles and subluxations in her neck.

The nerves that control muscles in your arms and hands and allow you to type a letter come out of your spine at the lower part of your neck. Many cases of carpal tunnel syndrome have their origins in this area, because pinched nerves in the neck create dis-ease in the wrists, which contain seven bones called *carpals*.

The carpal bones in your wrists are stacked in rows, with an opening between them—the *carpal tunnel*—through which nerves pass on their way from your neck and arms into your hands and fingers. If they are not receiving proper nerve flow, when your wrists are put under constant stress the bones move out of their normal position, pinching the nerves in the wrists and producing painful symptoms. In Claire's case we realigned the bones in her neck and wrists, and within a few weeks she was working pain-free. In addition, she was sleeping better and reported having more energy.

With computers cropping up in our homes and businesses faster than rabbits at a fur ranch, carpal tunnel syndrome is becoming epidemic. Many of these cases could be prevented if a trip to the chiropractor were included with a computer's standard software.

The best proof that pain from subluxations can take years to develop are children suffering from pinched nerves. We see this in our clinic every day, where 25 percent of our patients are under the age of fifteen. Very few two- and three-year-olds come in saying, "Dr. McGill, my neck hurts." Excluding accidents ("Tommy was jumping on the trampoline and landed on Karen's head. Can I bring them in?"), most of these children are seen because of posture problems, headaches, chronic ear infections, colic, asthma, sinus problems, or bedwetting. With the exception of headaches and traumas, their subluxations aren't causing pain, yet their bodies aren't working correctly. When we relieve the pressure from their nerves, their bodies work better.

OLD TIMES

Blocks in our bodies cause problems other than pain. For example, clench your hand into a tight fist. Can you feel how much more energy tight muscles use than those that are relaxed? Blocks are energy sinkholes, gobbling up vitality we could use in other areas of life.

Besides draining energy, blocks make us old before our time. Your biological age is simply a measure of how well your body works, compared to those of people of other ages. A key factor in figuring biological age is flexibility. A loss of flexibility accompanies any misalignment in the body. As your bones shift out of their normal position, they stop moving correctly. The bones often jam and begin sending out pain signals that cause muscle spasms in the area. Every day in practice I see longtime chiropractic patients in their forties and fifties with more flexible spines than new patients in their twenties and thirties. They may be older, but in some important respects they're actually younger.

Along with other problems, blocks can bring us down mentally and emotionally, because if your body isn't performing well, it's hard to think clearly or stay positive.

BLIND SIGHT

Right now you may be asking yourself, "Why haven't I ever heard any of this from my medical doctor?" Good question! The fact is, medical doctors know as much about most chiropractic as chiropractors know about prescription drugs, which is very little. Most doctors have never been to a chiropractor, never talked to a chiropractor, and, if they have been exposed to the subject of chiropractic in their schooling, have heard all the negative myths that earlier generations of doctors were led to believe out of ignorance.

For example, several months ago a new medical doctor opened an office not far from my chiropractic clinic. My brother-in-law, an airline pilot, went to him for a flight physical. He suggested I meet the doctor, who had just received his discharge from the military and was eager to make contacts in our area.

I invited the M.D., a former flight surgeon, to lunch. He was a very pleasant and intelligent man who seemed truly concerned about his patients. We started talking shop, and he asked me the sorts of cases I typically saw. I noted that about 30 percent of my patients came to me to get rid of their headaches.

"Really?" he said in amazement. "What could you do for someone who has headaches?"

Medical doctors are taught that misaligned bones in the spine rarely pinch nerves, because bones need to move a great deal before affecting nerve function. What they've only recently begun to learn is that the bones of a joint need only move a small amount to create abnormal nerve flow.

For example, once a joint becomes misaligned, receptors in it start sending signals to the brain reporting the problem. The brain then sends signals to the muscles around the joint, causing muscles to tighten in an effort to pull the misplaced bones back into position. Without this natural reflex, bones would stay out of alignment.

Sometimes, however, the joint doesn't go back into its proper position. You now have a block: the joint is sending out distress signals, and muscles in the area are in spasm. As other nerve impulses pass through the area on their way to or from the brain, their information becomes distorted. Once again the result is less-than-perfect function.

If you've read this book up to this point, you know more about chiropractic than most medical doctors do. This sounds outrageous, but it's true, so don't be surprised if your medical doctor doesn't diagnose blocks to the free flow of nerve impulses in your body.

SURVIVAL GUIDE

Besides wondering why medical doctors don't recognize the damage blocks create, you may be wondering why your nervous system responds to overload in a way that's so detrimental to your health. The answer is that our nervous systems often adapt our bodies to stress in the short term in a way that's less than beneficial in the long run.

For example, several years ago my father was shucking oysters when his knife slipped and the blade ran through his hand. At the hospital he received enough stitches to make a shirt, but after his hand healed, he was still left with a thick, jagged scar. Why did this happen? Why do you heal with scar tissue when you're cut, rather than with the kind of skin that was there before your injury?

Your body has a built-in survival mechanism that wants wounds to heal as fast as possible, to prevent infection. It uses scar tissue for this, which can be laid down much more quickly than "normal" skin. But scar tissue is "cheap" compared to the skin that was there before. It's inflexible and more prone to tearing, and when it's put under pressure, it tugs on the normal tissue around it, which can cause pain, itching, and other discomfort. Scar tissue helps prevent infection, but it leaves you in less-than-perfect shape.

Blocks work the same way. Though you function less than perfectly with them, you may not have been able to withstand the physical, emotional, mental, or chemical forces that originally assaulted your nervous system.

Most blocks dissolve soon after their job is done. In other words, when the overload situation passes, our bodies return to normal. If our bodies couldn't fix most misalignments and tight muscles, we would very quickly become sickly, stiff, and susceptible to disease. Simply getting enough rest is often enough to let tight muscles relax, and certain movements can be used by the body to realign itself. Have you ever turned your head or bent over and heard a pop or a click in your neck or back? Often this is your body realigning itself.

Sometimes your body can't realign itself, and blocks stay put. That's when chiropractic comes into play. The practice of chiropractic and the exercises in this book are designed to give your body the movement it needs to realign your spine and loosen your spasmed muscles.

REELING FROM THE YEARS

Physical, emotional, mental, and chemical stresses can be like wrecking balls, relentlessly pounding at your nervous system. If you don't reinforce your body and mind against assault, your nervous system can become overloaded, producing blocks. By creating parts of us that are inflexible and rigid, where life doesn't flow, blocks deaden us. As time goes on, they accumulate in our bodies. We take them on as baggage as we go through life, so that by the time we reach our sixties and seventies, large parts of our bodies are functioning at less than maximum potential.

Many of the examples in this book are taken from patients suffering from physical overload (car accidents, falling down stairs, and so on). This is because most people who seek out chiropractic care have developed symptoms related to physical traumas. But emotional, mental, and chemical stresses are common causes of nervous system overload as well. Just because you have never experienced an accident doesn't mean your headaches or back pains aren't being caused by the inability of your nervous system to function correctly.

The most common symptoms produced by blocks are headaches, neck pain, backaches, and feelings of anxiety and depression, but many other health problems are directly linked to our inability to cope with overload.

In the rest of this book you'll learn how to dramatically decrease overload's effects by removing blocks from your body and toning your nervous system.

4

THE SUNNY SIDE WAKE-UP ROUTINE

[conditioning your nervous system against overload]

At one time there were gypsies in places like Romania, Bulgaria, and Transylvania. They didn't have villages of their own, but traveled in caravans from town to town, camping out in the deep, dark forests.

The gypsies lived a good life, but they had a problem. There were bands of wolves that also roamed the forests. The wolves would prey on the gypsies. They'd come into camp and steal food, bite children, and generally be a pain in the goulash. The gypsies had a terrible time fighting off these wolves.

Then one night a band of gypsies built a big bonfire in the center of their camp. They noticed that with this bonfire burning, the wolves didn't attack. They said to themselves, "Hey, maybe we can start building bonfires instead of fighting wolves!" They did, and their lives became much better.

While this parable is a bit of an exaggeration, it teaches us an important lesson about health:

Rather than waiting for health problems to attack, we need to concentrate on building the inner bonfire of health burning within each of us. The best time to start is tomorrow morning, with a simple morning wake-up routine.

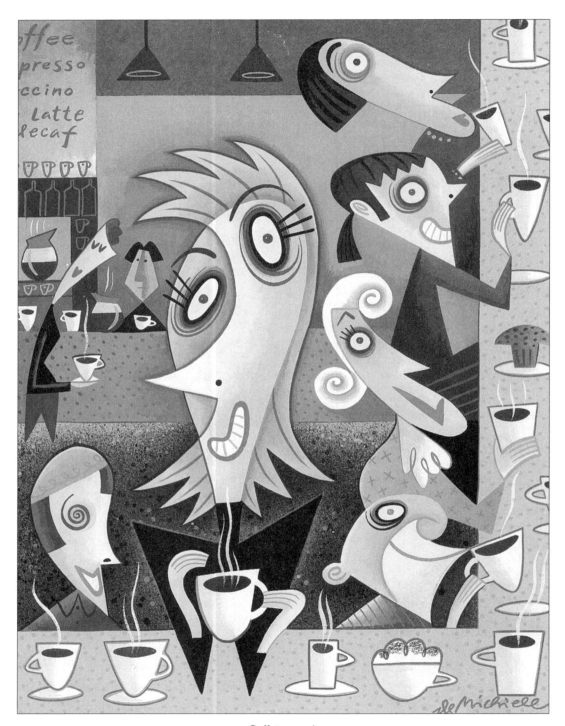

Caffeine rush

SNOOZING AND LOSING

Many of us go through a morning ritual in which we drag ourselves out of bed, then shock our nervous systems into alertness with coffee, soft drinks, or sugary sweets.

Dawn is a typical example. She came to me suffering from migraine headaches, which tended to come on late in the day, during her last few hours at work.

During our initial consultation, Dawn also complained that she always felt tired. She looked tired, with dark circles under her eyes and a yellowish tinge to her skin. I would have guessed she was in her mid-thirties, but in reading her chart I saw that she'd recently celebrated her twenty-eighth birthday.

She was having trouble sleeping, sometimes because of headaches, and sometimes because, as she put it, "I can't turn my mind off." In talking with Dawn, I learned that when her alarm clock sounded in the morning, she awoke feeling almost as tired as she had when she went to sleep. She usually hit the "snooze" button several times before dragging herself to the bathroom, where she relied on a hot shower and the strong scent of deodorant soap to wipe the thick cobwebs from her eyes.

She drank two cups of coffee with breakfast, which usually consisted of sugary cereal. At lunch she often stopped for a 32-ounce, caffeine-loaded fountain soda at a convenience store. She sometimes drank two or more of these huge drinks during the day.

Dawn's morning wake-up routine wasn't only contributing to her headaches, it was wearing down her body faster than a milling stone grinding wheat.

THE ENERGY ROLLER COASTER

Energy and alertness can be "bought" with coffee, soda, and sweets, but at a high price.

For example, one reason the caffeine in coffee and soda is so effective is that it rushes into your bloodstream and blocks the action of chemicals that normally slow down your nervous system. It's as if you cut the brake lines on a car traveling down a mountain. Nerves fire more rapidly. Your

51

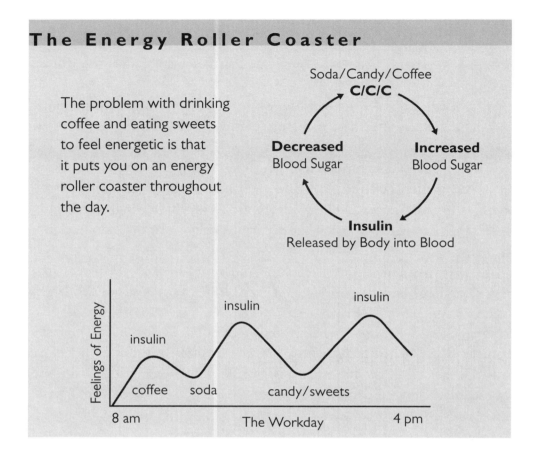

The Energy Roller Coaster

The problem with drinking coffee and eating sweets to feel energetic is that it puts you on an energy roller coaster throughout the day.

Soda/Candy/Coffee
C/C/C

Decreased
Blood Sugar

Increased
Blood Sugar

Insulin
Released by Body into Blood

Feelings of Energy

insulin

insulin

insulin

coffee   soda   candy/sweets

8 am   The Workday   4 pm

body roars to life, with increased blood pressure, a faster heart rate, and speedier breathing (although these effects vary among individuals).

The problem is that your body wasn't meant to race at such a fast pace, which may explain coffee and soda drinkers' increased susceptibility to sleeplessness, restlessness, and "burned out" feelings.

Sugary foods pose other problems. Many foods, including fruit and bread, have basically the same chemical composition as candy. However, the sugar in a banana is gradually absorbed into your bloodstream. Refined sugar, on the other hand, rushes into your blood, creating high levels of blood sugar, which, if uncontrolled, can lead to all kinds of nasty health problems. To bring blood sugar down, your pancreas, a gland tucked underneath your stomach, pours the chemical insulin into your bloodstream. Insulin takes sugar from your blood and transfers it into your body's cells. Excess sugar is then turned into shiny globs of fat, which is stored throughout your body.

Some experts think that after years of straining to keep your blood from turning into a candy store, the pancreas eventually "burns out." It loses the ability to produce adequate insulin, and you develop diabetes, a disease in which your body can't produce sufficient amounts of the chemical.

Apart from the wear and tear on their bodies, Dawn and millions like her who rely on coffee and sweets for energy put themselves on an energy roller coaster every day. In the morning they drink coffee or soda containing caffeine, sending nerve impulses crackling through their bodies like those big sparks Dr. Frankenstein used to bring his monster to life. In addition, the sugar in the coffee, soda, or breakfast cereal dumps into the bloodstream, increasing blood sugar. *Voilà!* Instant energy.

But within a few hours the caffeine wears off, blood sugar drops, and Dawn, feeling as though someone has cut the wires to her battery, heads for the coffeepot, soda machine, or snack bar. She gets another "fix," which lifts her to another energy peak. Her body responds by bringing the unnatural blood sugar level down. Another energy pothole. And so it goes throughout the day.

Getting on such an energy roller coaster every day leads to mood and productivity swings and robs us of the chance to develop a strong, reliable, inner abundance of energy.

WAKE UP, TUNE IN

How can you build an inner bonfire of health? The answer is to enliven your body with a morning wake-up routine. The following system is designed to improve your eyesight, sense of smell, and breathing capacity. Also included are ways to release tension from your jaws and tongue, and the muscles of your face. The system even includes specific steps for maximizing your kidney function and digestion.

Think of this wake-up ritual as a tonic you can take every morning that will, over time, build an incredibly strong yet flexible nervous system. Many of the longest-lived people on earth start their days with such routines, taking a few moments to get in touch with the natural power of their bodies to heal and function at a high level.

The Sunny Side Wake-up Routine

Approximate Workout Time: 15 minutes

The following routine is done in bed when you first awaken. Just prop a pillow comfortably behind your back, and you're ready to start. Of course, you don't have to do it in bed. It works great as a warm-up before a regular morning exercise and stretching routine, or anytime you feel like refreshing yourself, in which case you can do the routine in a chair or cross-legged on the floor.

As you move through the routine take deep, slow breaths (see "Belly Breathing" on page 128). You'll start with your eyes and work down your body, ending at your feet.

The Eyes

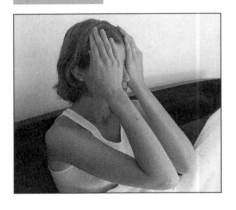

- Rub your hands together for about ten seconds, until they begin to warm.

- When you've generated some heat, use your hands to cup your eyes. Feel the warmth soak into your eyes for a few seconds.

- Repeat three times.

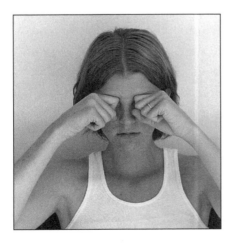

- Make fists and rub the sides of your index fingers together, again generating some heat.

- Using the middle knuckles of your index fingers, rub them over the top ridges of your eye sockets. Start near the bridge of your nose and move outward. Make three quick strokes from the inside out.

- Rub the index fingers together again, and make three strokes on the undersides of your eye sockets.

- It's time to stretch the muscles responsible for moving your eyes. Keeping your head straight and still, look up and to the right. You should feel the muscles around your eyes stretch, just as if you were stretching a leg or an arm.

- Keep looking up and to the right. Don't try to focus your eyes, just feel the stretch. Continue for about ten seconds.

- Repeat the exercise, looking up and to the left.

- Repeat again, looking down and to the left.

- Repeat again, looking down and to the right.

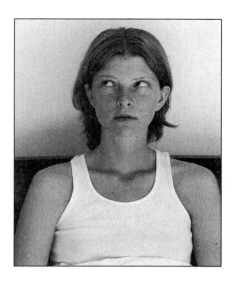

- Now move your eyes in a circle. Start by looking straight up, then slowly move your eyes clockwise to the right, down, left, and up. Complete three circles.

- Repeat, moving your eyes counterclockwise.

- Finally, close your eyes and, using the tips of your fingers, gently massage your eyeballs with four slow, soft strokes, moving from the bridge of your nose to the outer corners of your eyes.

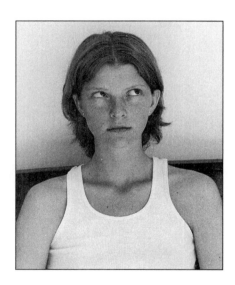

Though it sounds a little complicated, the whole eye segment takes about two minutes, and its effects are dramatic. I've used these exercises many times at rest stops when driving long distances, and have been amazed at their refreshing effect.

Jaw, Tongue, Lips, Teeth, Mouth, and Throat

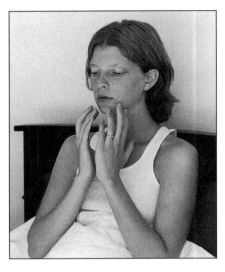

- Open your hands, spread your fingers, and, using the tips of your fingers and thumbs, tap your jaws, starting just below the ear and working down to the chin.

- Tap around the mouth and between the nose and lips, then move back up to just below the ears. Tap for ten to fifteen seconds.

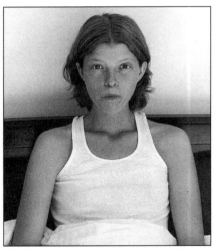

- Now, with your mouth closed, move your tongue between your teeth and lips in a clockwise motion nine times. Repeat the motion counterclockwise nine times.

- Move the tongue inside the teeth and "wash" the inside of the teeth, nine times clockwise and nine times counterclockwise.

- Note: your tongue may not be toned enough to make nine sweeps. If this is the case, start with four sweeps and build up to nine at your own pace.

After all this tongue movement, you will have built up a healthy supply of saliva in your mouth. Swallow this in three small sips. (Some people may find the thought of this offensive. Try not to skip it; it's one of those ancient Oriental secrets of good health that seem to have surprisingly positive effects on well-being.)

Finally, click your teeth together gently twenty-one times. Do this fast, feeling the vibrations shake into your gums.

The jaw/tongue movements outlined above loosen some of the most-used muscles and joints in the body. They are especially helpful to those who suffer from TMJ (temporomandibular joint) problems, in which the jaw joints ache and click.

Ears, Scalp, and Cerebellum

■ Now take your ears between your thumbs and forefingers and gently massage them, starting at the tops and working down to the lobes. Take about ten seconds to give these headsets to the world of sound a good tune-up.

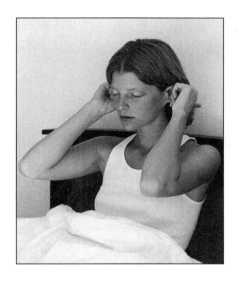

■ Next, again open your palms and spread your fingers, making your hands into "claws." Press your fingertips lightly against your forehead and vigorously run them over your scalp toward the back of your skull. Move your hands so that you cover the entire scalp.

■ Do forty-eight strokes. This will increase circulation to the scalp, improving your alertness.

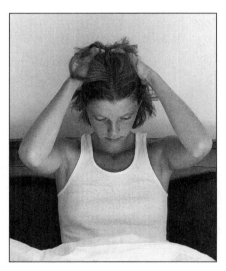

■ Now cup your ears with the palms of your hands. Using the index fingers to first resist and then release the middle fingers, flick the middle fingers against the back of your skull.

■ This maneuver is called "banging the heavenly drum" in certain martial-arts traditions. It stimulates activity within the cerebellum, the part of your brain responsible for balance and coordination.

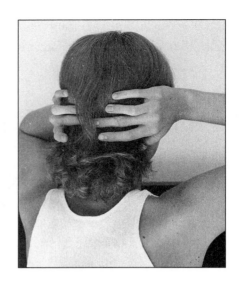

Combined with the eye exercises outlined above, "banging the heavenly drum" is an excellent tool to use whenever you need to quickly refocus your attention. It's especially helpful to use as a pick-me-up during long periods of concentration, such as reading a difficult book or working for hours at a computer.

The Chest

■ Making a fist with whichever hand feels more comfortable, lay your arm over your chest and raise and lower your fist in a thumping action against your chest. Do this as hard as is comfortable. Repeat twenty-one times.

Besides sending vibrations into the chest to stimulate air flow within the lungs, this maneuver stimulates the thymus gland. Tucked underneath our breastbone, this gland helps the body manufacture antibodies that strengthen the immune system.

The Kidneys

- Sitting up straight, cup your hands and place the palms of your hands on your back, about six to ten inches up from your waist. Rub your back with an up-and-down motion.

- Rub for ten seconds, heating the area. This gentle movement stimulates kidney function and is helpful in eliminating the waste products of digestion that have accumulated overnight.

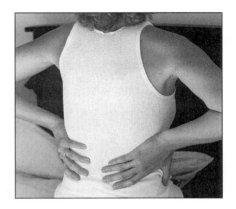

The Intestines and Colon

- Rub your hands together, generating heat. Cup whichever hand is most comfortable and place it on the skin just underneath your navel.

- Rub briskly in a clockwise motion eighty-one times, generating warmth. This movement awakens the powerful energy center called *tan t'ien* in traditional Chinese medicine.

- Now, using your index and middle fingers, find a spot just below and slightly to the outside of your kneecap, midway between the center of your shin and the outside of your leg (you may feel a shallow groove running along the outside of your skin—your fingers fit in this groove). Gently press in with your fingers and rub in a circular motion twenty-one times on both legs; this stimulates a point on your body related to digestive health.

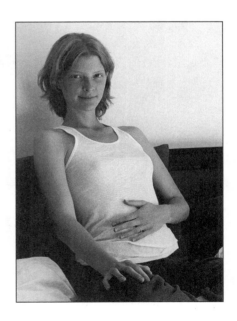

The Feet

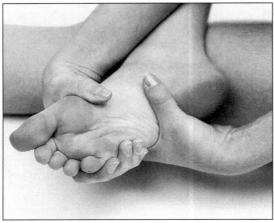

■ To complete the wake-up routine, gently grasp your right foot with both hands and rub the foot in a wringing motion, starting with the heel/ankle and working your way up toward the toes.

■ When the entire foot has been rubbed, push the toes forward, then bend them back.

■ Repeat with the left foot.

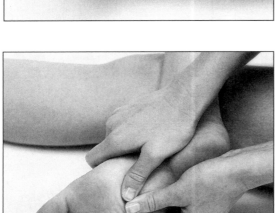

■ If you have extra time, use your thumbs to gently massage the undersides of your feet, searching for any tender spots and spending twenty seconds or so massaging these tender areas. Massaging the feet not only prepares them for the rigors of pounding the pavement, but also stimulates the functions of many internal organs.

■ To finish your wake-up routine, close your eyes, take in a deep, slow breath . . . then slowly blow it out through your nose.

Take your shower, or continue to build your inner bonfire of health with some morning exercises such as the ones outlined in the next three chapters.

5

POSING PROBLEMS

[posture's dramatic impact on your health]

"Stand up straight!" mothers beg their slumping children, and for good reason. Posture affects our appearance and health in remarkable ways.

For example, last year a teenager came to see me complaining of neck and back pain. David said he'd always been sickly, spending several weeks each year hospitalized with pneumonia. Each day he swallowed blood pressure medication, though his doctors were at a loss to explain why his blood pressure remained high.

An X ray of this fifteen-year-old's back showed his spine dramatically curved to the side, a condition known as scoliosis. Scoliosis causes many postural problems, ranging from uneven hips and shoulders to a "hunchback."

David's spine was curved most in the upper back, where nerves exit and travel to the lungs and heart. I felt that many of his health problems stemmed from pinched nerves along his spine, and I told him that along with getting rid of his back pain, there was a good chance we could keep him out of the hospital. I didn't mention chiropractic's success at lowering blood pressure in many patients.

David progressed rapidly, his pain fading in about two weeks. During his third week of care he visited his "blood pressure doctor." Remarkably,

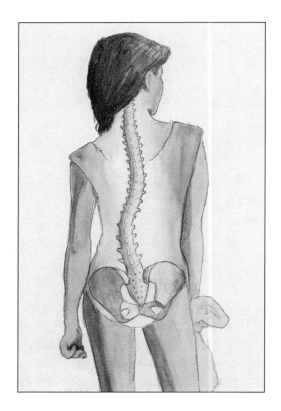

Congenital Problems
Spinal problems you may have had from birth may make you more susceptible to spinal degeneration because your spinal structures have been stressed from the beginning.

his readings had dropped a full ten points, from $^{145}/_{100}$ to $^{135}/_{90}$. He's now medication-free, and his lungs are working fine. This is a surprisingly common example of a patient's posture compromising heart and lung function. By relieving the nerve pressure caused by David's posture, we changed his health for the better.

CURVES AHEAD

To "stand up straight," you need a spine with four front-to-back curves, two curving toward the front, and two curving toward the back.

Your spine's curves keep you functioning in the fast lane. Your neck and low back curve forward, helping support your head squarely over your shoulders and your torso over your hips. The middle spine slopes backward, making room for your heart and lungs. Likewise your tailbone, also curving back, gives your bladder and colon room to fill, and in women it eases a baby's trip from womb to delivery room (though not as much as most women would like).

The Curves in Your Spine

If you could see your spine from the side, you would notice that your spine curves naturally at its upper, middle, and lower segments. These curves are designed to support the weight of your upper body and provide flexibility.

Your **upper spine** (cervical curve) supports the weight of your head, which is held in place with muscles and ligaments.

Your **middle spine** (thoracic curve) supports the weight of your upper body.

Your **lower spine** (lumbar curve) supports the weight of your trunk and upper body and provides a stable foundation for your other two curves.

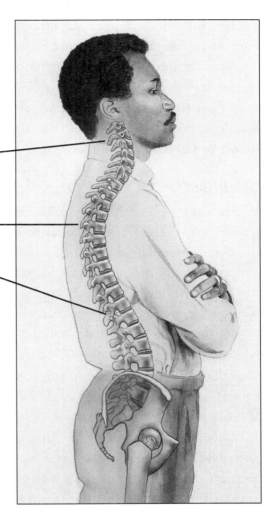

PULLING YOUR OWN STRINGS

Your spine keeps you standing straight, but it couldn't do its job without your "antigravity muscles." These muscles are at the front and back of your body. For example, the *erector spinae* (erect spine) group are thick muscles on both sides of your spine running from your hips to the back of your head.

To imagine how these muscles work, picture a belt loop at the small of your back, a pulley at the back of your head, and a rope running from the belt loop through the pulley. The erectors work as if someone were standing behind you, pulling this rope, arching you backward.

In front, another set of antigravity muscles, the abdominals, run from your lower rib cage to your pelvis; when working they pull you forward.

The antigravity muscles are important because most of your body's weight is in front of your spine, giving you a tendency to fall forward. Like tent ropes pulling against each other, the muscles on the front and back of the body keep us upright. If they stopped working, we'd crumple to the floor like puppets without strings.

GIFT GIVING

When your spine is correctly curved and your antigravity muscles are working smoothly, a natural alignment develops—your head balanced over your shoulders, hips, knees, and ankles. This is good overall posture, with your body balanced front-to-back and side-to-side.

Good overall posture is important, but many postural problems show up in isolated areas of our bodies.

For example, when I was talking with Jenny, a new patient, about her headaches and back pain, I noticed her head cocked to the right, like someone trying to eavesdrop on a conversation. In Jenny's case this was caused by a shift of the first bone in her neck to the left, which tilted her head in the opposite direction.

One person's head might tilt to the right, another may have bones in her mid-back shifted out of their normal alignment. As individual as fingerprints, these postural problems are often tracks left by nervous system overload. Blocks in the body, they result from misaligned bones and abnormally tight or loose muscles.

If you develop postural problems your body performs at less than peak efficiency. I see this frequently in children with "foot flair," a condition in which one of their hips rotates in, shifting the foot outward. They have a harder time running, and their athletic ability suffers. (Foot flair is usually remedied easily by realigning the hips. In fact, most children respond to this sort of care in less than a month.)

HIDDEN AGENDAS

Most postural problems aren't as obvious as a hunchback or a rotated hip. In fact, like your heartbeat, your temperature, and 300,000 or so other functions constantly taking place in your body, how you hold yourself is usually controlled subconsciously by your nervous system. When your nervous system becomes overloaded, the blocks formed in your body wreak havoc on your posture.

THE POSTURE OF STRESS

Carrie is the mother of six young children. Years of caring for four girls and two boys while trying to stretch the family budget have taken their toll. Overweight and overstressed, at thirty-two she already has a large hump at the top of her spine, the kind often seen in seventy- and eighty-year-old women. Her head hangs off the front of her shoulders as if a bag of cement were roped to it.

Carrie is suffering from "the posture of stress," which is just the opposite of a relaxed pose. What's relaxed? Think of those advertisements for Caribbean resorts, where a bronzed couple lies side by side on a white sand beach, blue-green water lapping lazily behind them. The models are melting over their lounge chairs. Their heads are tilted back as they drink in the calm moment. They might even have their hands behind their heads, really letting the sun soak into their chests and bellies. That's relaxed.

What would happen to this couple's posture if rebel soldiers taking control of the island started bombing the beach? The couple would probably throw themselves facedown in the sand, curling into balls, their arms over their heads. If they tried to run for cover, they'd hunch over, heads bent down.

One theory says stress bends us forward because such a stance protects our bodies' most vulnerable parts, including the head, neck, belly, and sexual organs. Other animals with spines walk on all fours, their vital parts protected from above by their backs, from the sides by ribs, arms, and legs, and from below by the ground.

The posture of stress probably developed to protect the body in times of physical danger. As time went on, however, our nervous systems learned to bend us forward in times of *any* perceived danger, physical or mental.

If you've been to Caribbean resorts, you may have noticed that some

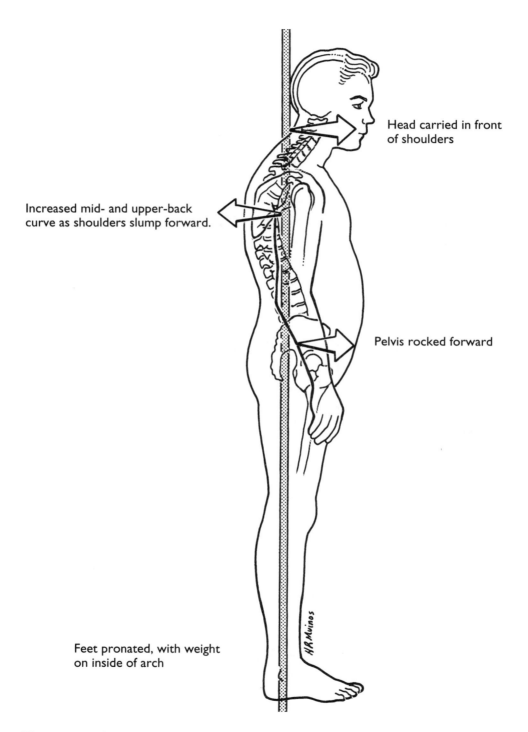

Head carried in front
of shoulders

Increased mid- and upper-back
curve as shoulders slump forward.

Pelvis rocked forward

Feet pronated, with weight
on inside of arch

The posture of stress causes lasting changes in the way we hold ourselves.

tourists don't look all that relaxed in their lounge chairs. The problem is that *repeated stresses overload your nervous system and affect every muscle in your body, every second of the day.*

Once we're overloaded, blocks form and we stay in the posture of stress until our nervous systems calm. Unfortunately, many of us lack the tools to "de-stress," with disastrous results. Anxiety, headaches, and decreased energy result when excess excitation becomes trapped in our bodies, winding us tighter than spools of thread.

ANXIOUS MOMENTS

I love bookstores, but for several years a bully named Anxiety wouldn't let me enjoy them. I'd walk into a book emporium feeling terrific, excited by the prospect of thumbing through the latest releases. Within minutes, however, Anxiety made his presence felt. My neck muscles started twisting into rope-tight bands. My heart began pounding, and I felt light-headed and sick to my stomach. I didn't know why. Anxiety attacked like lightning out of a blue sky. Subconscious ideas I wasn't aware of caused my mind to tighten my body's muscles.

These same physical sensations paralyze many people when flying, getting into elevators, or driving over bridges. While different situations make different people anxious, virtually 100 percent of the time we're conscious of our unease because of *feelings* in our bodies, usually in the form of tight muscles.

Stress research shows that the mind/muscle connection also works in the opposite direction; like college students calling home for money, your muscles are always sending messages to your brain to let it know how things are going. *If your body's muscles are tense due to a physical, mental, emotional, or chemical overload, they send signals to your brain that are interpreted as anxiety.* Soon a vicious cycle develops. The body tells the brain it's tense, and the brain reacts by tensing the body.

A person in the posture of stress is especially susceptible. They are like the proverbial camel carrying a huge load of straw, wobbling back and forth on shaky legs. Just as another straw breaks the camel's back, one disturbing thought or bit of excess stimulation creates anxiety.

In my case, my anxiety about bookstores faded after a chiropractor realigned my spine. My body relaxed, so my mind could handle more disturbing thoughts before triggering anxious feelings.

Many of my patients report similar stories. I once asked a mortgage broker about changes in his mental attitude under chiropractic care. He explained that he'd always had a "really short fuse":

"I used to jump down people's throats at the office about any little thing," he said. "But since I've been coming here, it takes a lot for me to fly off the handle."

SUPPORTING CAST

While nervous system overload produces the posture of stress and is at the root of many anxiety attacks, it also causes a staggering number of headaches. Here's how: When the posture of stress bends us forward, the neck's natural curve is eliminated. As the head, weighing eight to twelve pounds, drops forward, the spine no longer supports it and the neck muscles now must strain to keep the head over the shoulders.

In the short term this isn't a problem. But as the posture of stress continues, the neck muscles become tense and tight. Sometimes, as in Carrie's case, these muscles can become quite large.

Tense, tight neck muscles are involved in 90 percent of all common headaches, producing them in two ways. One is through pinched nerves, the other through the "spasm-pain-spasm" cycle.

SQUEEZE PLAY

When neck muscles tighten inappropriately, they often tug the first and second bones of the neck out of their normal positions. (This can be a chicken-or-egg situation, because bones can also become misaligned through physical trauma, causing muscles to tighten.) As the bones become misaligned they put pressure on nearby nerves that are responsible for controlling the function of blood vessels and muscles on the scalp.

Soon scalp muscles spasm and blood vessels constrict. Often the headaches created by pinched nerves start at the base of the skull, intensifying as they move onto the head and wrap around to the temples.

Tension Headache
Tension headaches are the most common kind of headache you can get. Although stress and fatigue can make them worse, or trigger the onset of pain, a tension headache often starts with misaligned vertebrae. This misalignment may irritate a spinal nerve, setting in motion other physical problems, like tightening muscles, and causing the steady "viselike" pain of a tension headache.

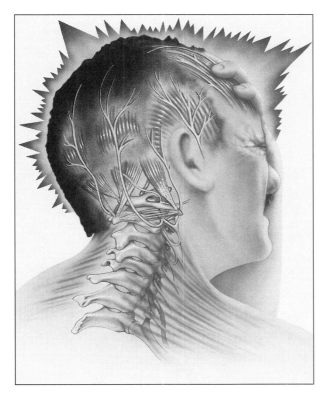

1. **Poor posture** over time or spinal injuries lead to misalignment, which is worsened by stress.

2. A **misaligned vertebra** irritates a **spinal nerve,** which sends "warning" signals to surrounding neck muscles.

3. The **neck muscles** then tighten up (spasm) to protect your misaligned vertebra. This irritates underlying nerves in your neck.

4. These **irritated nerves** send warning signals up to your head muscles. In response, they tighten up suddenly.

5. These **tightening muscles** create a chain reaction of spasm and pain encircling your head—a tension headache.

Chiropractic "cures" headaches by relieving nerve pressure so that muscles and blood vessels can function normally.

TIME BOMBS

Just as common as the headaches let loose by pinched nerves are those set into motion by the spasm-pain-spasm cycle, which begins when neck muscles stay tense. In this unnatural state, small pockets of extremely tight muscle develop, which we call **trigger points.**

Trigger points are dime-size land mines waiting to explode in the neck and head. When tense muscles are physically or mentally stressed, trigger points within them activate. This throws the muscle tissue surrounding the point into painful spasm. Pain signals race to the brain, and the brain, in a protective reflex, increases muscle tension even more.

Bonnie Prudden describes this sequence in her book *Pain Erasure*:

> *A trigger point lies quiet in a muscle until the physical and emotional climate is right, and then it "fires." Its firing throws the muscle into spasm. This causes pain, and the autonomic nervous system . . . sends more spasm to the affected area to protect it against whatever is threatening.*
>
> *When the spasm sent by the nervous system reaches the designated area, it further tightens the spasm already present. That hurts! Another pain message shoots back to headquarters predictably followed by yet more spasm. This phenomenon is called "splinting." We now have a spasm-pain-spasm effect, and until it is broken the pain will continue unabated, and as the pain continues, so will the splinting. This shortens the muscles and holds them in a foreshortened condition, which not only causes pain but interferes with function, posture, and balance.*

The most hazardous trigger points are the ones located right beneath the skull. As these fire, muscles on the head and neck spasm, creating headaches. When examining a patient suffering from chronic headaches I often find pinched nerves and trigger points together in an area right beneath the back of the skull. They go together, but like the chicken and the egg, it's hard to know which came first.

BREATH CONTROL

While posture problems caused by nervous system overload land a one-two punch with anxiety and headaches, they also dramatically deflate our energy by robbing our oxygen supply. As Philip Smith notes in his book, *Total Breathing*:

> *Each emotion has a unique breathing pattern all its own. If we are tense and afraid . . . the chest and stomach area tend to collapse in, thus preventing the full inflation of the entire lung area . . . we tend to breathe in*

*a quick and shallow fashion in an attempt to provide the lungs with suf-
ficient oxygen.*

An easy way to feel how a stressed posture obstructs your breathing is
to do this test:

Drop your head and shoulders forward in a slump, so that your chin
rests on or near your chest. Try taking a deep breath through your nose.
Notice how noisy the breath is, and how the air going into your lungs
stops at the top of your chest. Now hold your head up and your shoulders
back. Take another breath. Can you feel how the air streams in more easily, flowing freely toward the bottom of your rib cage?

MUSCLE BOUND

With the power to dish out anxiety, headaches, and low energy faster than
McDonald's serves up french fries, it's not surprising that posture problems also cause chaos with our muscles.

For example, we said the antigravity muscles were like tent ropes.
Actually, they're much more dynamic. When you're walking, your brain
changes the tone, or tightness, of your antigravity muscles hundreds of
times each minute to keep your head, spine, and pelvis in the best possible
alignment.

If your spine becomes misaligned, your antigravity muscles do their
best to pull you back into shape. They tense, they tighten, and, like
Winston Churchill in his famous line, they never, never, never quit.
Unfortunately such persistence propagates problems. Most people walk
into my office carrying backs riddled with extremely tight, painful muscles
straining to realign their spines.

Don came in recently complaining of upper back pain. On examination, I found his right hip positioned one quarter inch higher than his left.
Because the legs attach to the hips, every time he took a step, his body
tilted to the right.

Our brains program our muscles to keep us walking upright, our eyes
level with the horizon. Don's brain righted his posture by tightening muscles along the upper back. But the muscles strained so hard righting the

wrong of a high hip that they began crying out in pain. Once we leveled his hips, Don's upper back relaxed for the first time in years.

SAME OLD GRIND

Bones and joints are affected by poor posture, too. A smooth, shock-absorbing material called cartilage covers the ends of bones and keeps them from grinding against each other. If bones remain aligned, their cartilage-covered ends move as smoothly as marbles rolling on a polished floor.

If bones lose their proper alignment, their cartilage-covered ends begin grinding. Inflammation sets in, and soon the cartilage starts breaking down. Ultimately, misalignments lead to one of the most common health problems of our time, degenerative arthritis.

Arthritis simply means "inflammation of a joint" (from the Latin *arthra,* meaning "joint," and *itis,* meaning "inflammation"). Unfortunately, many physicians label any long-standing joint pain "arthritis." Often they don't recognize the role of misalignments in causing the problem, or that restoring proper alignment may dramatically improve the condition.

Recently Virginia, a spunky eighty-three-year-old, was referred to me by her sister. She had injured her left shoulder many years before, when she was thrown from a horse. Over the years the shoulder had developed arthritis. The pain was so bad that for three weeks Virginia had spent her nights pacing the floor, sobbing from the intense ache.

Her medical doctor told her, "It's arthritis. There's nothing you can do except take an anti-inflammatory." But the pills hadn't worked. On her first visit I realigned the bones making up Virgina's shoulder joint. That night she slept through the entire night for the first time in months.

BONE TIRED

Bones in the spine degenerate when misaligned, too. Perhaps the best examples are misalignments created by whiplash-type auto accident injuries.

In a classic whiplash, a car is hit from behind. The driver and passengers of the struck car accelerate forward, their heads snapping back. Then the car suddenly stops and their heads snap forward. It's estimated that about 30 percent of all drivers will suffer a whiplash during their lives.

Whiplash injuries produce misalignments throughout the body, but

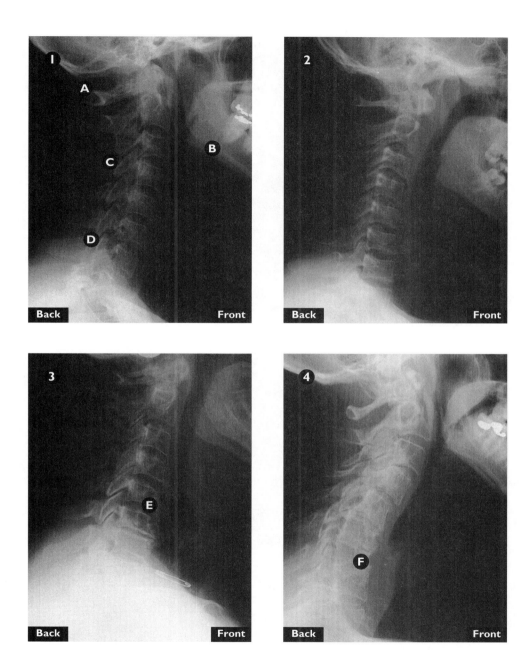

Reversed aging. These X rays are side-views of the neck's seven vertebrae. To orient yourself: A is at the back of your skull. B: bottom of the jaw. C: back of the neck. D: base of the neck, where it joins the shoulders. The neck should curve forward (1). Trauma or other stress can cause the neck's normal curve to reverse (2). Now bones degenerate, losing their normal square shape as bone "spurs" develop (3/E). As degeneration continues, bones fuse together (4/F).

The Powerful Force of Whiplash
Whiplash turns your head's weight into a powerful force, hurling your neck past its normal range of motion. In the typical whiplash injury, your head is whipped backward, injuring muscles, ligaments, disks, and other structures. As your head whips forward, its speed doubles, increasing the force on your neck. If your head is turned to the side, injury is often more severe.

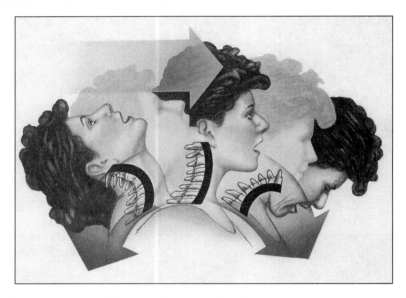

Before impact, your neck's natural curve is aligned.

Your head whips backward, exaggerating your neck's curve.

Your head snaps forward, reversing your neck's natural curve.

most damage occurs in the neck, which often loses its natural curve. Now when the person twists, bends, or turns, these normal movements are forced upon misaligned bones. Often the bones start pinching nerves, and the person develops headaches, neck pain, and tingling and numbness in the arms and fingers. Inflammation also develops, and the slow process of degeneration begins, leading to arthritis.

Recently a thirty-seven-year-old man came into my office complaining of sharp, intense neck pain that shot down his shoulders and into his arms. On his X rays I was surprised to see a tidal wave of degenerative arthritis in his neck. The fourth, fifth, and sixth cervical vertebrae had degenerated so badly they'd developed bone "spurs." These are small, horn-shaped bits of bone that eventually grow together and fuse the spine into a rigid structure. It's thought that they are the body's method of stabilizing areas of the spine where degeneration changes normal movement.

The man said he'd been in a "real bad" motorcycle accident as a teenager, and had been living with neck pain for fifteen years. It took several months to get his neck working properly. Once we did, however, I believe we stopped the slow process of degeneration.

PAIN AND POSTURE RELIEF

The most common cause of pain in the neck and back is chronically tight muscles, often brought on by misaligned bones pinching on nerves in the area.

Once a muscle tightens and stays tight, several things happen that lead to pain. First, the muscle begins working much harder than normal. You saw this before when you clenched your fist and felt how hard your muscles work when they're tight. All that effort produces chemical waste in the muscles.

If you hold your fist clenched for a period of time, you'll notice the blood draining out of it. That's because, as the muscles tighten, they squeeze blood from the arteries and capillaries in the area. Now you've created a recipe for pain: The muscles are tight, producing waste, but there's not enough blood flow to wash the waste away.

As waste products accumulate, they begin irritating the muscles, causing pain. When the brain receives pain signals, it increases muscle tension in the area, decreasing blood flow further and adding more pain. If the situation is allowed to continue, the area becomes a site that's continually painful.

Sometimes we develop tight areas in our bodies, but they're not tight enough to produce discomfort. Then we get stressed, and the added stress creates enough additional muscle tension to produce pain. When you relax a bit, the pain stops, but that area of your body remains tight and tense, waiting to produce more pain the next time you're stressed.

Exercises for the neck and back help relieve pain by loosening the muscles, allowing more blood to flow through them, eliminating the waste products of muscular effort and allowing misaligned bones to gain better alignment, increasing nerve flow to the muscles.

The neck pain relief exercises outlined below are aimed at relieving stress in the neck and shoulders, the areas most prone to problems caused by poor posture. If you are suffering from headaches or pain and tension in the neck and shoulders, concentrate on this easy, ten-minute routine. For best results, do it twice a day, morning and evening. If your time is limited, it's best to do the exercises in the morning, after taking a warm shower. You can also do the Self-Massage portion of the routine through-out the day. Once you're out of pain, pick two or three exercises from the routine to do daily in order to stay pain free.

Please note that although this book is designed to help you develop near-perfect nervous system function, there's no substitute for your chiro-practor's advice. You'll obtain the best and fastest results by using this book in conjunction with the chiropractor of your choice, who can act as a personal health coach. At the end of this chapter, and each of the fol-lowing chapters, you'll find space for your chiropractor to write down his or her recommendations concerning the exercises and techniques outlined. These "prescription pads" allow your chiropractor to tailor the ideas pre-sented in this book to your individual needs.

Neck Pain Relief
Approximate workout time: 10 minutes

The Shoulder Shrug

Many people instinctively shrug their shoulders to relieve tension in this area. The key to making shoulder shrugs work for you is to do them slowly, with proper breathing. Here's how:

■ Stand or sit up straight.

■ Taking a long, slow, deep breath into your belly, begin to raise your shoulders.

■ Continue inhaling as your shoulders come up as high as they can stretch, and as you push the shoulders back.

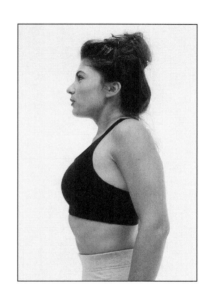

■ When your shoulders are pushed as far up and back as they will comfortably stretch, begin to exhale.

■ As you slowly let all your breath out, push your shoulders down and then forward and up.

■ As you begin to inhale again, repeat the up-and-back movements, and exhale as you push the shoulders down and forward.

■ Exaggerate the movements as much as possible without causing yourself pain. Don't speed up. The slower the better. Do four repetitions.

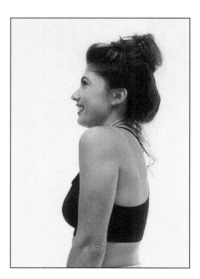

The Shoulder Shrug, Part 2

Now that your shoulders and neck are warmed up, it's time to increase your stretching movements.

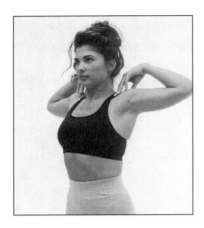

■ Place your fingertips on your shoulders. Now, as you inhale, slowly raise your elbows up and back. Begin to exhale as you continue to rotate your elbows in a wide circle, bringing them toward the ground.

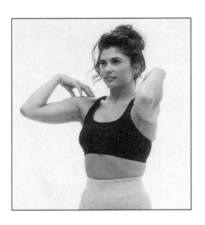

■ Continue to exhale as you lift your elbows up and forward, so that your elbows come together in front of your chest.

■ Note: Your breath should be let out all the way as your elbows meet in front of your chest. Begin inhaling again as you bring the elbows up toward the ceiling, out to the sides, and back. Repeat four times.

The Reader

- Start by holding your hands in front of you, palms at shoulder height and facing you as if you were reading a book.

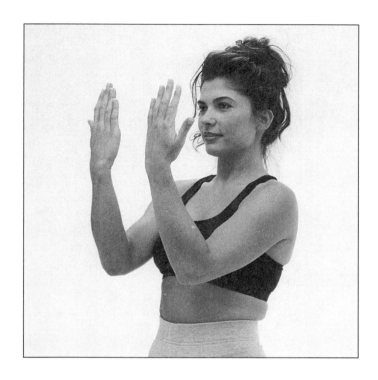

- As you inhale deeply, raise your arms and keep your eyes on your "book," so that your head arches back. Don't arch your back. You should feel a good stretch under your arms and across your chest.

- With your arms upstretched, hold the pose and your breath for a count of two.

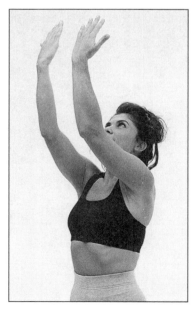

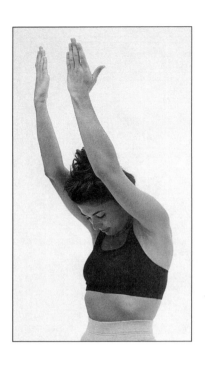

■ Now exhale fully and slowly drop your head toward your chest, letting your head hang limp as you exhale fully.

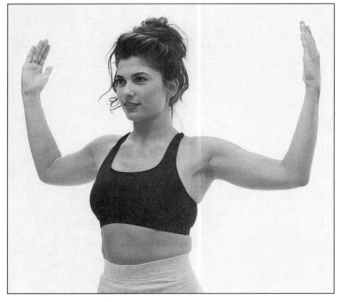

■ Take another breath in and, keeping your arms in an L shape, press your elbows back so that your chest fully stretches and expands. Hold for a count of two.

■ Now breathe out and pretend you're diving off a diving board, bringing both arms as far out in front of your body as you can while letting your head drop to your chest. Hold for a count of two.

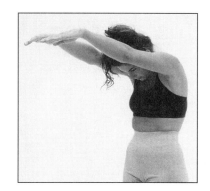

■ Inhaling, come back to the starting position.

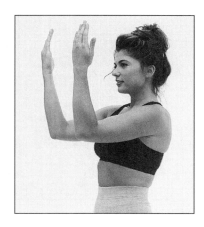

■ To finish this exercise, exhale and let your chin drop to your chest. Rest for a count of two.

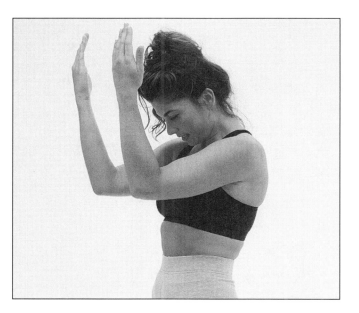

Repeat this exercise four times. To start your second repetition, raise your head to the starting position, inhaling as you raise your arms.

Trigger Fingers

The explosive trigger points in your neck and on your skull that are at the root of so many "tension" headaches can be defused with this exercise.

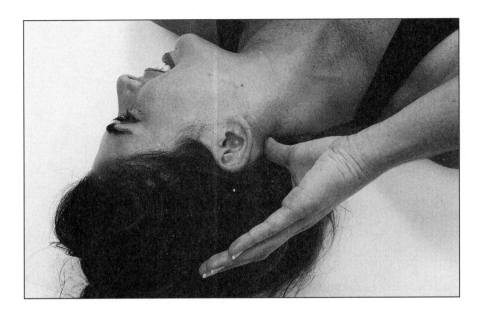

- Start by lying on your back. Get comfortable.

- Turn your head to the left. With your thumb, press into the base of your skull, just behind the right ear.

- Press along the groove right beneath your skull until you find a particularly tight spot. It is likely a trigger point. Press firmly into the spot. This will cause some pain; don't overdo it. Hold for a full count of seven, counting "one thousand one, one thousand two," and so on.

- Move along toward the middle of the skull, erasing trigger points as you go.

- Turn your head to the right and do the left side. Try erasing trigger points once each day for two weeks and thereafter, whenever your neck muscles begin tightening.

Self-Massage

You may be lucky enough to have a mate or loved one who is always willing to massage your sore neck and shoulders. . . .

I didn't think so. Even if you had someone like that, it still would be nice to have a good massage at your fingertips. You do! Here's the best way to rub the kinks out of your own neck and shoulders:

- Cup your right hand and move it to the left shoulder.

- Starting at the base of your neck, begin squeezing the muscles there. Work your way out toward the end of the shoulder, squeezing each section two or three times.

- Now work your way back up toward the neck.

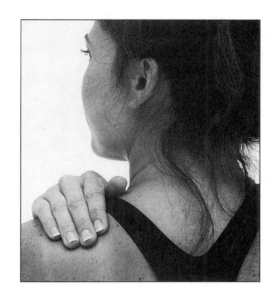

- When you've finished, flatten your hand and press your fingers together so that you can use the tips of your fingers to dig deep into your muscles.

- Start at the base of the neck and, using a circular motion, dig the tips of your fingers into the tops and backs of your shoulder muscles.

- Keep digging as you move out to the end of your shoulder, concentrating on any tight spots.

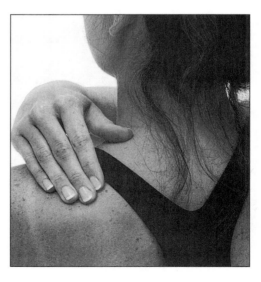

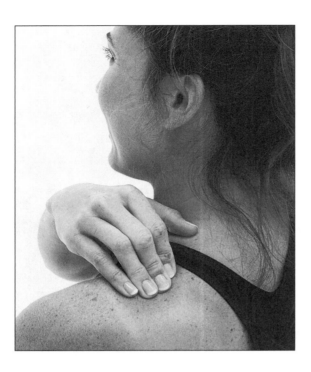

■ Now find the tightest spot and, using the tips of your fingers, drag that area forward toward your chest, releasing it when your fingers slide over the top of the shoulder.

■ Repeat on the left.

The Perfect Posture Program
Approximate workout time: 10 minutes

To rid our bodies of the blocks caused by nervous system overload, we must get out of the posture of stress. If our neck muscles are chronically tight, we need to loosen them. If trauma has changed our posture for the worse, we need to reverse those effects. We may never achieve perfect posture, but by working at it, we can calm our nervous systems. As we do so, our bodies begin functioning at a higher level.

The following exercises will help rid your body of blocks while realigning it, opening up nerve pathways long shut off. A combination of ancient wisdom and modern science, the Perfect Posture Program will get you standing tall and healthy again. If you have growing children, the exercises will let you stop complaining about slumping shoulders and drooping stances and let you start training your children to stand in the healthiest way possible.

The Ball Bearing

This exercise reverses the forward-bending posture of stress by bending your body backward over a small plastic ball. As you do this, you may hear "pops" or "clicks" in your spine. This is a good sign, indicating your spine is adjusting itself to a new, healthier posture. You may also notice a dramatic increase in the amount of air you can inhale.

I recommend using a ten-inch ball, available for a few dollars in most toy departments. If you experience discomfort, try a six-inch ball until your back becomes accustomed to its new flexibility.

As with all exercises aimed at tuning your nervous system, breathing correctly is extremely important when doing this exercise. When doing any exercise in this book, breathe slowly through your nose. Concentrate on your breath. Notice how it flows in and out of your body as you exercise. As you exhale, feel your muscles become more and more relaxed.

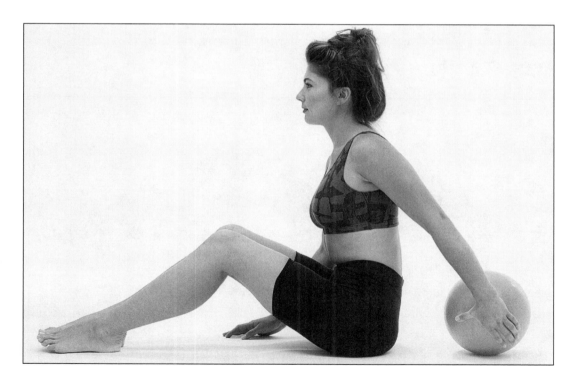

■ Sit comfortably on the floor and position your ball so that when you lie back, the ball rests between your shoulder blades.

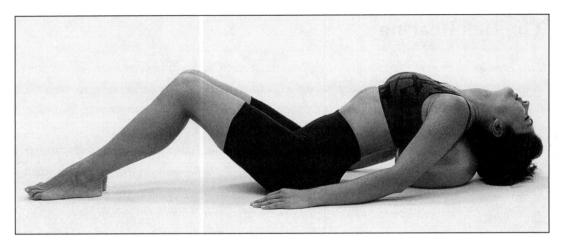

- Take a breath; as you slowly exhale, lie back on the ball.

- Let yourself relax, and feel your body sink down toward the floor. Imagine that you're at the beach, that your body is made of wax, and that you're melting over a warm beach ball on the sand.

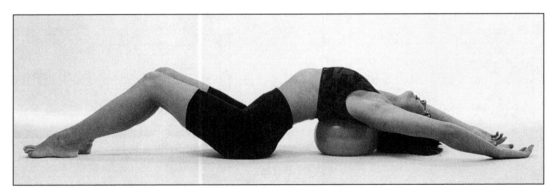

- If it's comfortable, raise your arms over your head for more of a stretch.

The Ball Bearing is a short routine—five slow, deep breaths, and you're through. It only takes a minute, but goes a long way toward reinvigorating your posture and energy level.

The Back Loop

This exercise is an antidote to civilization. As civilized people, most of our daily activities bend us forward. The most devastating habit is sitting, because virtually all of us sit in a way that bends us forward. (I'm reminded of this as I sit at my computer terminal, trying not to slouch after four hours of typing.) At school, at desk jobs, on soft furniture at home, in car seats— we're forever bent over. Is it any wonder that nervous system overload has such an easy time trapping us into an awkward, forward-bent posture?

The Back Loop reverses forward bending. The key is that it utilizes the back's erector muscles, which become stretched and weak in most members of our slumping society.

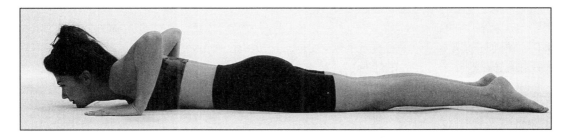

■ Lie facedown on the floor, with your hands resting close to your shoulders. Raise yourself up slightly so you can comfortably touch your chin to the floor.

■ Take a deep breath, and as you slowly blow it out, raise your torso up off the floor while looking straight ahead.

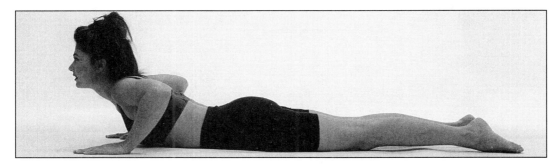

■ Try not to push up with your arms; use your back muscles as much as possible.

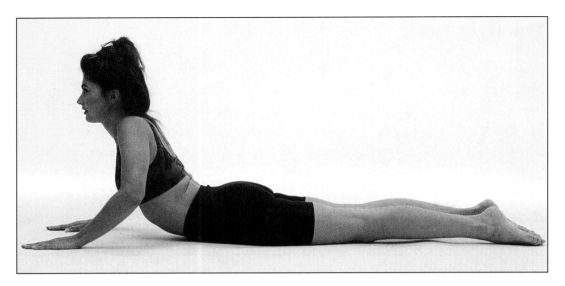

- Come up only as high as is comfortable. Because we use these muscles so little, it's best to take it easy on our first Back Loops. As your back muscles get stronger, you'll be able to lift higher off the ground.

- Do five Back Loops. On your fifth attempt, hold your highest position and slowly breathe in and out through your nose. The first time you attempt this won't be easy; you may only be able to hold the position for a few seconds.

- Be gentle with yourself, and increase the last part of the exercise until you can hold the position and slowly breathe in and out three times.

The Wall Slide

Tired of slouching? The Wall Slide is designed to counteract our slumping postures. It's easy to do, and all you need is a wall (or door) to lean against.

The "slide" stretches the curves in the low back, mid-back, and neck, refreshing the muscles along the spine while aligning ears, shoulders, hips, and ankles.

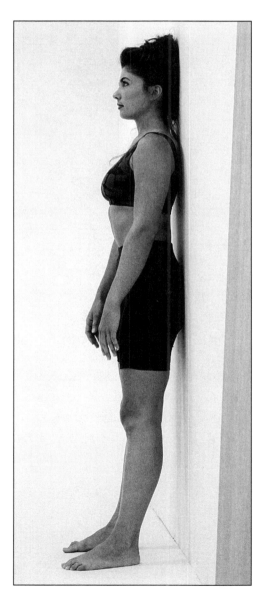

- Stand with your feet shoulder-width apart, about six inches out from a wall (door). Lean back.

- As you take a deep breath in, bend your knees and slide down until your knees are comfortably bent.

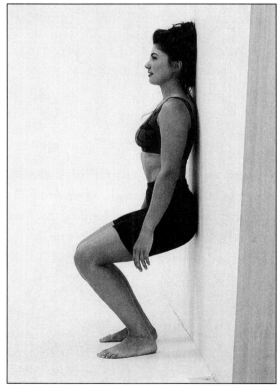

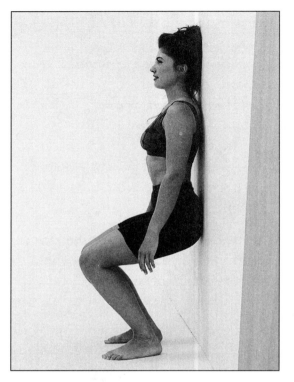 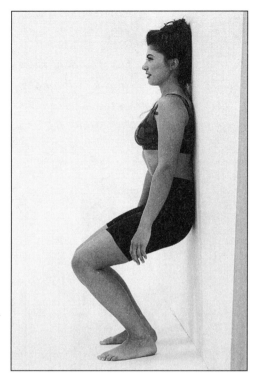

■ Now press the lower part of your back, your shoulders, and the back of your neck against the wall.

■ After you are flat against the wall, exhale slowly while sliding up. (You may not be able to get your back completely flat against the wall; try your best, but don't strain.)

Do the Wall Slide four times. This is also an excellent exercise to do throughout the day to refresh your spine and posture. When finished with a set of slides, keep your erect posture and step away from the wall, maintaining this near-perfect stance for up to thirty seconds.

The Wall Slide helps remind our nervous systems what it's like to enjoy good posture, conditioning our bodies into a more youthful stance.

The Chest Breath

This exercise opens the chest and tones the muscles between your shoulder blades, which are crucial to maintaining an upright posture.

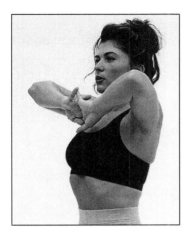

■ Sit or stand erect, your chin level with the floor, your hands and elbows just below shoulder level, with your fingers intertwined and your palms facing away from you. The backs of your hands should be resting on your chest.

■ Take a deep breath, and tighten the muscles between your shoulder blades. Feel your chest expand.

■ As you exhale, let your back muscles relax and push your hands out in front of you as far as possible. Feel the muscles along your arms and around your shoulders stretch as you let out all the air.

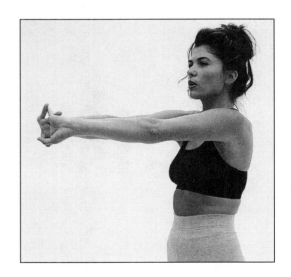

■ Hold for a count of two, then inhale again, tightening the back muscles, filling your chest.

■ Repeat eight times.

If you work at a desk all day, this is an excellent exercise to relieve muscle tension and help keep you from slumping.

91

The Seagull

This routine helps combat the rounded shoulders that so many of us develop from bending forward all day. You'll be strengthening the muscles at the tops and backs of your shoulders in order to pull your torso up and back.

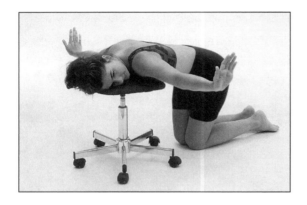

- While kneeling, lay your head and the top of your chest on a chair or low table.

- Extend your arms straight out from your shoulders, with your hands pointed up toward the ceiling. Be sure to hold the hands in this position, or you won't be able to isolate the proper muscles you want to strengthen.

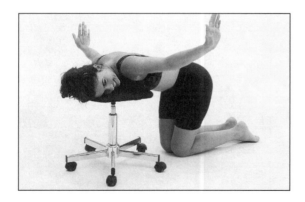

- Breathe normally and, keeping your hands pointed, raise your arms slowly up toward the ceiling, raising them as far as is comfortable; then slowly let your arms down.

Try not to cheat by using your arm muscles; concentrate on tightening the muscles across the tops of your shoulders in order to raise the arms. Repeat ten times, then turn your head and do another set of ten.

The Turtle/Turtle, Part 2

Few people realize how important their necks are to their well-being. Connecting your head to your body, the neck contains more nerves per square inch than any other body part.

As we've seen, if the neck is bent forward in the posture of stress, the muscles at the back of the neck naturally become strained trying to keep the head over the shoulders. But there is more to the story.

When your neck becomes flexed forward, the spinal cord stretches, becoming overly excited. Nerves along the spine now fire more readily, causing muscles along the back to tighten.

The Turtle helps keep and restore the neck's natural curve, decreasing the stress on the muscles at the back of the neck and relaxing the entire spinal cord.

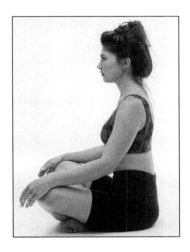

■ Sit up straight in a chair or car seat. Level your chin and eyes with the horizon—you should not be looking up or down, but straight ahead.

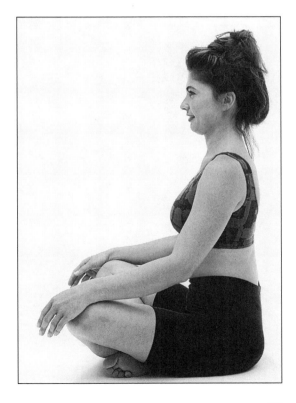

■ Bring your chin back, keeping it parallel to the floor.

Caution: This exercise will create sore muscles if done too strenuously. Do the exercise slowly, and STOP if you experience pain. Also, the natural tendency is to tuck the chin, but don't do this. Retract the neck back over the shoulders as you exhale. Do this ten times.

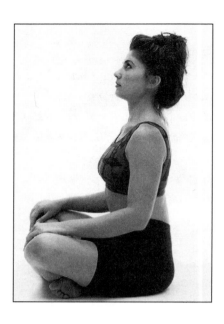

■ The Turtle, Part 2 is an even more powerful neck toner. As with the Turtle, retract your neck over your shoulders.

■ Now, with your neck retracted, lift your chin one to two inches up toward the ceiling. Your natural tendency will be to tilt your head back over your shoulders, but avoid doing this. Keep the back of your head as stationary as possible while you lift your chin. This motion isolates the muscles you need to work. Repeat ten times. Use caution not to strain the muscles at the back of your neck.

If you are in a chair, at the end of your Turtle and Turtle 2 exercises, take a deep breath in; as you exhale, release a long sigh, letting your chin drop to your chest. Feel the muscles at the back of your neck get a good stretch.

My Chiropractor's Advice:

6

PELVIC POWER

[tuning your nervous system from the bottom up]

Perry and I were looking at an X ray of his low back, taken minutes before. The thirty-nine-year-old refrigeration repair technician had experienced low-back pain for most of his adult life, especially when lifting and bending. Lately he was having trouble getting up from chairs and his favorite couch, and had started to walk, as he put it, "like an old man," bent over at the waist.

"We call your pelvis a primary area of your spine, because it's the foundation on which your spine rests," I was saying, explaining why chiropractors put so much emphasis on the part of your body that includes your belly in front, your buttocks in back, and contains your low back, tailbone, and hips.

Using a pencil, I drew a line on the film across the tops of Perry's hips. Then I marked the center of each bone in his low back.

"The line across the tops of your hips should be even with the floor, and the bones of your low back should be lined up nice and straight as we come up the film," I explained.

I asked Perry what he saw when he looked at his hips.

"The right one is higher," he said.

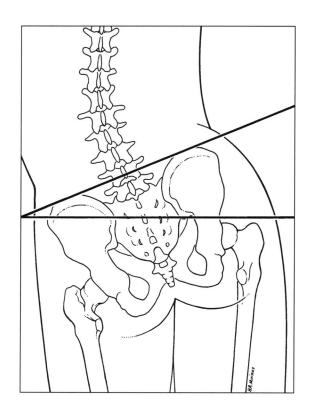

The Leaning Tower of Pisa Effect. Spinal misalignments often develop as a result of an unlevel pelvis.

"That's right," I agreed, noting that the right hip was about one quarter inch higher than the left, making the line connecting the two look like an off-balance teeter-totter. "If you were going to build your dream house, would you build it on a foundation that looked like that?" I asked.

As Perry shook his head and chuckled, I said, "Of course not, because when you built the second story, your windows and walls would be crooked! It works the same with your spine."

We turned our attention to the bones of his low back. Like a cupped left hand, they curved up and away from the high right hip.

"I call this the 'Leaning Tower of Pisa Effect,'" I said. "If your right hip is higher than your left, your low back usually curves to the left because it's resting on an uneven foundation. If your left hip is high, your low back usually curves to the right."

Like most people who suffer from low-back pain, Perry's spine contained subluxations (minor misalignments of the bones making up the spine). They "pinch" nerves and cause them to malfunction. Because the nerves aren't working correctly, dis-ease develops in the body, eventually leading to symptoms.

Like most patients, Perry wanted to know *how* his spine had gotten into such shape. I didn't have a ready answer. Perhaps as a boy he'd fallen off his bicycle or down some stairs. Maybe his low back became misaligned while playing sports. Perhaps at some point in his life he'd faced tremendous emotional problems, with the resulting muscle tension pulling bones out of alignment, where they became stuck. Unless someone comes in for treatment immediately after a trauma, it's usually impossible to say how misalignments in the low back first occurred; we don't know from day to day how our bodies react to the stresses we put them through.

Perry's muscles were also involved in his low-back pain. They were chronically tight from trying to realign his hips and the bones of his back. However it had become misaligned, Perry's back contained blocks to the free flow of nervous system energy, causing him problems.

POWER CENTER

If you want your body to be as powerful as a locomotive, you're going to need a pelvis that's as strong as a steam engine. Your largest muscles are located in this part of your body. They create tremendous internal forces. With every contraction of a pelvic muscle, your head, shoulders, arms, and legs all respond, as if someone shook the base of a tree and all its branches shuddered.

Since your whole upper body hangs from your spine, any pelvic movement is transferred to your chest, neck, head, and arms. Likewise, your legs attach into your hips. When your hips move, so do your legs. Pelvic movements act like earthquakes, sending out waves of energy to every other part of your body.

When they're working correctly, your pelvic and low-back muscles do most of the work as you get up, sit down, run, walk, bend, or twist. If they become tight, your body can develop decreased function as far away as your neck and ankles, in turn causing problems all the way to your fingertips and toes. Many so-called primitive peoples realized this, and developed dances and other practices to keep their hips and low backs loose and limber. The Hawaiian hula dances are a good example.

ALTERNATIVE ENERGY SOURCES

While the area between our bellies and buttocks has always been seen as powerful, many ancient health traditions recognize it as an energy center as well.

It's easy for us educated in Western science to understand how energy flows along nerves. This electrical energy is easily measured. There is a nonelectric energy in the body as well. It doesn't flow over nerves and, so far, hasn't been measured by scientific instruments. In traditional Chinese medicine it's called *ch'i* (pronounced "chee"), and means "life energy."

Ch'i is concentrated in the belly, and flows throughout the body along invisible pathways called meridians. When people go to acupuncturists and get stuck with needles, the physician is unblocking the flow of this invisible energy.

Unlike the majority of medical doctors, chiropractors have traditionally been open to the idea of a second energy system in the body. Many have recognized the validity of acupuncture and acupressure (a variation in which fingers are used instead of needles), and have incorporated these techniques into their practices. Some of the exercises at the end of this chapter, as well as part of chapter 4's "Sunny Side Wake-Up Routine" and chapter 8's "Dynamic Relaxer" exercise, are designed to influence your body's *ch'i* energy system.

BRAIN POOL

While some chiropractors explore the flow of *ch'i* energy, others are working with the flow of another substance crucial to your body's vitality.

It's long been known that a special liquid is contained within your skull and spine. It's called cerebrospinal fluid, or CSF. Like jellyfish in the ocean, your brain and spinal cord float in a sea of CSF.

In studying the spine, chiropractors have found that CSF flows in waves from the tailbone up the spine, and around the brain. This movement is powered by a "pump" located in the pelvis. As we breathe, our tailbones gently move forward and back, sending CSF flowing up and down our spines.

The brain and spinal cord dump waste products into the CSF, which carries them away. If your pelvis loses its normal motion and the natural flow of CSF is blocked, waste products can accumulate and decrease your nervous system's health.

BACK BITTEN

Linda was lifting a twenty-five-pound bag of fertilizer from the back of her pickup truck. As she pressed the bag against her chest and stepped away from the truck, she tripped over a small ledge and fell backward. As she caught herself, a sharp pain shot through her low back. When she got to our office, Linda was bent forward at the waist. When I asked her to bend backward, she came up about six inches before grimacing from the pain. With a little laugh, she said, "That's it. I can't believe it, but I can't go up any higher."

How to Lift

Most lifting injuries occur because we don't think before we hoist a heavy load. Before beginning a lift, plan on accomplishing five actions:

1. Bend your knees and lift with your legs. Transferring stress from your back to the large muscles of your legs is the best way to prevent injury.

2. Tighten your abdominal muscles. Tightening the "abs" transfers tension from your low back to your belly, forming a "girdle" of muscle around your waist that protects your back.

3. Get close to the object you're lifting. This helps your balance. Keeping the weight close to your center of gravity also transfers stress from your arms and back to your legs.

4. Avoid twisting while lifting. If you need to move an object to the right or left, keep your torso over your hips and feet and take several "baby steps" in the direction you need to go.

5. Keep your shoulders back. This will help keep your back straight, allowing its muscles to work most effectively.

Cheryl took advantage of a warm spring day to do some yard weeding. She spent several hours hunched over, pulling tough little plants up by the roots. One particularly stubborn dandelion just wouldn't come up. She positioned herself in a squat over the pesky plant and pulled with all her might. Something "gave" in her back. As she tried to stand up, she felt the bite of a muscle spasm rip into her side. After two days on a heating pad, she came into the clinic with a dull pain simmering in her low back. "I can't move an inch without it grabbing me," she said.

Linda and Cheryl were suffering from the two most common problems that cause back pain. In Linda's case, she'd jammed joints in her low back. Cheryl, on the other hand, had overextended herself and pulled muscles in the area.

When joints become misaligned, a potentially painful situation develops. Instead of sliding smoothly on each other, the bones catch, sending out sharp pain signals.

Linda's low-back joints jammed when she fell backward. Nerves within the joints began screaming while muscles around it tightened. Not only did her joints jam, but the bones making up the joints became misaligned. They started putting pressure on the nerves running from the spinal cord out into the body, again with painful consequences.

Pulled muscles are common in the low back because the area is often tight, tense, and prone to problems. When Cheryl put too much strain on her low-back muscles, they began to tear. As soon as her brain sensed this overexertion, it tensed her back muscles tighter than a miser's hold on his last penny, producing a pain so urgent that Cheryl had to stop damaging herself.

It's easy to understand how accidents and overexertion can hurt our backs. But many people live with sore, stiff low backs every day, without doing anything more strenuous than getting out of bed in the morning. Our lifestyles are often at the root of these low-back problems.

STOOPED AND CONQUERED

In the last chapter we talked about how slumped postures can create neck problems. Bending forward doesn't help your low back, either. Why does a back massage feel so good? Because our back muscles are usually extremely tight, fighting to hold us up while we insist on slumping forward! Unfortunately, few of our daily activities exercise the low-back muscles to keep them flexible and strong. Instead they become weak yet tight, creating fertile soil in which nervous system overload can grow.

CHAIRPERSONS

Another enemy of your low back is the chair you're sitting in. Alexander Mathias, inventor of the Alexander Technique, a posture realignment method, called chairs "the worst instrument of our civilization." He observed that chairs compress our low back and cause stiff, cramped leg muscles.

Balanced act. Taking a break from chairs eases tension in your lower back.

Studies have shown there are far fewer back problems in cultures where people squat on the ground rather than sit in chairs. X-ray studies of such "squatters" show their chairless lifestyles help produce good posture.

Chairs create another problem as well. As we sit day after day, our leg muscles become tight and our knees inflexible. When we stand, our knees lock. Your knees act as shock absorbers when they're bent, but if you walk or stand with locked knees, all the stress is transferred to your low back.

I see this in my office every day, where, after their spinal tune-up, patients are asked to change their treatment table's sterilized paper. To do this, they need to bend down. At first, virtually all of them keep their knees locked when they bend down to change the paper. After I teach them to keep their knees bent, many people report far less back strain in and out of the office.

WEIGHTY ISSUES

It's hard to avoid sitting in chairs. But many of us create similar strains on our low backs by carrying extra pounds in our bellies. As a person's belly gets bigger, the curve in his low back increases. It's as if the low back were being dragged forward. This tends to jam joints in the area, pushing the person toward pain attacks. When we lose pounds, or tighten our stomachs through exercise, we relieve pressure on our low backs.

How to Sit at a Desk

To sit more comfortably at a desk:

1. Roll up a small bath towel so it's about five inches wide. Tuck this roll into the curve of your low back to support you while you sit. Experiment with the diameter of the roll, finding a size that's just right. "Lumbar supports" (cushions shaped to conform to the shape of your low back and give it support) work even better. They're available from your chiropractor, at stores like K mart and Wal-mart, or from orthopedic supply stores.

2. Taking time every now and then to exercise the neck and shoulders helps prevent them from tightening. Chapter 5's Shoulder Shrug, Shoulder Shrug Part 2, Turtle, Turtle Part 2, and Chest Breath are all excellent exercises you can do at your desk. Take a three-minute break every hour to do four repetitions of each exercise. During breaks, get up and try four repetitions of the Wall Slide from Chapter 6.

3. Sit close to your desk, and push your buttocks against the back of your chair to prevent yourself from slouching.

4. If typing, use a "copy stand," a device used to hold documents in an upright position, rather than looking down at papers laid flat on your desk.

5. A small box (about six inches high) can be placed under your desk. Rest one or both feet on this box periodically to help relieve tension on your low back.

EMOTIONAL ROOTS

As we've seen, emotions can become rooted in our muscles. Just as we tend to hold anger in our jaws, certain emotions seem to be associated with our pelvic muscles. Specifically, the powerful emotions surrounding our sexuality can affect the way we hold this part of our body.

For example, psychologists studying how our bodies reflect our mental attitudes find that some people hold their pelvises back in a tense posture.

They say such people may be afraid of expressing the depth of their sexual feelings. By "holding back" the pelvis, they repress their sexuality. If the pelvis is held forward, with flat buttocks, sexual energy isn't allowed to build up.

Psychologists say decreased sexual pleasure and performance may result from chronically tight pelvic muscles. During sex there should be pleasurable, spontaneous, and involuntary movements throughout the body. Free movement of the pelvis is best, where it can rock forward and back without restriction. Blocks can put a lock on your body's ability to move in an easy, uninhibited way. Sex becomes more mechanical. Relieving pelvic blocks can increase sexual pleasure and performance.

BASEMENT BLUES

When blocks take hold in our bellies, low backs, and buttocks, pain can become our constant, unwanted companion. Studies show that more than 80 percent of us will experience significant low-back pain at some point in our lives. It's the most common reason for lost work time and the second most common reason (behind respiratory infections) for a trip to the doctor.

Discovering the cause of a person's low-back pain is a challenge for any physician. One reason is that both joint and muscle problems can cause similar complaints. For example, *sciatica* is the medical term for pain running down the leg. A misaligned bone in the low back that's pinching a nerve can cause sciatica. But so can a tight buttock muscle or a jammed pelvic joint. And anyone who's ever suffered from a so-called slipped disk knows the leg pain it can produce. (Disks are fluid-filled sacks sandwiched between the bones of your spine. When a disk "slips," it bulges out—imagine a hamburger sliding partly out of its bun. The bulge can press on nerves coming out of the spinal cord and running down the legs, creating pain so intense it brings grown men to tears.)

The complexity of low-back pain is reflected in its treatment. Not long ago, low-back surgeries were fairly popular, even though many of them achieved only 50-percent success rates. The growing acceptance of chiropractic and improvements in other nonsurgical methods of treatment have decreased the number of such surgeries, while new surgical techniques have improved the success of necessary operations.

Among all the treatments for low-back pain, chiropractic has been shown to be the most effective, because it focuses on improving the *functioning* of your back.

FOCUSING ON FUNCTION

Your low back is a marvelous blend of strength and flexibility. Like a tree trunk, it should be strong. Like bamboo, it should bend. The "Get-Out-of-Back-Pain" and "Pelvic Power" routines given below are geared toward ridding your back of blocks while increasing its flexibility and strength. They're designed to make your low back work better as a whole, rather than treating specific joint, muscle, nerve, or disk problems.

Stretching and strengthening exercises are used to remove blocks, decrease joint and muscle stress, and improve the flow of CSF within your spine and skull. You may also notice more pleasure and better performance during sex.

If your low back is in pain, naturally you should concentrate on the pain-relief exercises first. Also, set up an appointment with the chiropractor of your choice. She or he will act as a coach, training this area of your body to be the power generator it was designed to be.

The Get-Out-of-Back-Pain Routine
Approximate workout time: 10 minutes

The Knee Pull

■ Lie on your back, preferably on the floor. (You can do this exercise in bed, but the results will be less dramatic.)

■ Raise your knees up in the air and grab them with your hands. If you've lifted your head off the ground in order to reach your knees, let the head drop back down.

■ Take a deep breath in; as you exhale, let your shoulders and neck muscles relax.

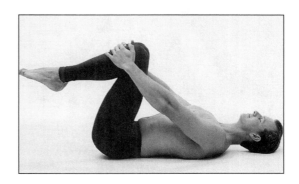

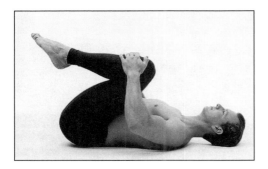

■ Inhale, and as you let your breath out, pull your knees gently toward your chest. You should feel a good stretch in the muscles of your low back. Don't strain.

■ When you get to the point where you start to feel pain, stop and let the rest of your breath out.

■ Breathe in again as you let your knees drop away from your chest. Go slowly! Don't try to force your sore back muscles to stretch too much. Let them relax, and try to feel the tension drain out of them. Repeat five times.

The Deep Tilt

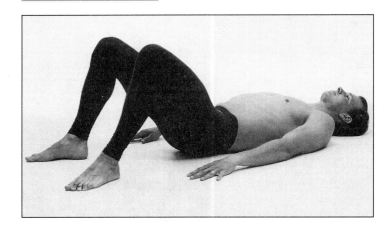

■ Begin by lying on the floor with your knees bent. Let your shoulders and waist relax. Take a deep breath in.

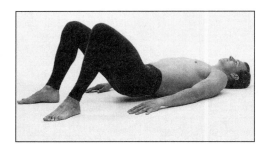

■ Then, as you exhale, keep the small of your back pressed against the floor and tilt your waist up, trying to bring the tops of your hips up toward your chin. To do this you'll need to contract your stomach and buttock muscles. Do this motion slowly and smoothly.

■ Inhale as you let your waist drop back down toward the floor.

■ Exhale and repeat the tilting motion. Repeat five times.

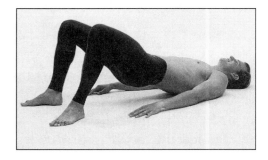

■ As your muscles get stronger and your pain fades, you may want to gently lift your buttocks off the floor as you tilt up, increasing the benefit of this exercise.

The Side-to-Side

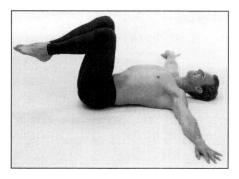

■ Begin by lying on the floor, your knees bent, feet flat on the floor, arms at shoulder height and outstretched to the sides.

■ Raise your knees toward your chin so that your feet come up and your heels rest on or near the backs of your thighs. Take a deep breath in.

■ As you slowly exhale, let your chin drop to the left while your knees drop to the right. Keep your knees together; drop them only as far as is comfortable.

■ Inhale as you return to the starting position.

■ As you exhale, drop your chin to the right as your knees fall to the left.

■ Inhale, returning to the starting position. Repeat three times to each side.

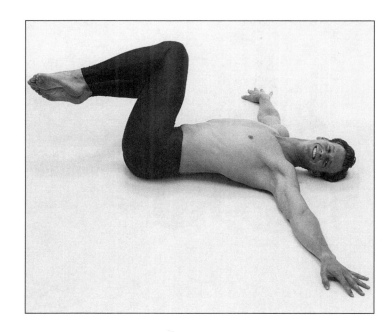

The Bicycle

This is an excellent exercise for people who have tight hamstrings—the large muscles at the backs of the thighs. Tight hamstrings, which are common in people who sit at a desk most of the day, often contribute to low-back pain.

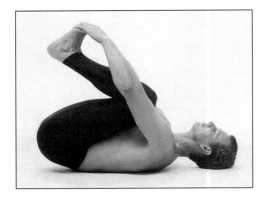

- Begin the Bicycle by lying on your back. Raise your knees up to your chest and grab your toes or the tips of your shoes.

- You may have to stretch and raise your head off the floor to get hold of your feet. Once you do, relax and let your head drop back to the floor.

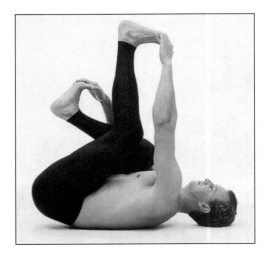

- Start with the left leg and push it out, attempting to straighten the leg. Stop when the leg won't extend anymore. Count "One."

- As you bring the left leg back toward your chest, push the right leg out, again stretching to its limit. Count "Two."

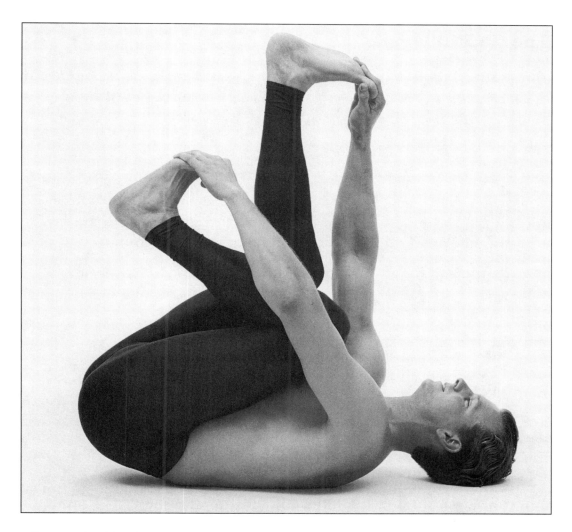

- Repeat the bicycle motion to a count of fifty, push-ing out first with one leg, then with the other.

- Keep your head on the floor, and don't strain. It may take several weeks before you are able to extend your legs out fully. Once you get to that point, add even more stretch by grabbing the *sides* of your feet or your shoes rather than the toes.

The Back Builder

The only way to strengthen our back muscles is to use them to bend us back. The Back Builder does just that. However, do not attempt this exercise until you are almost completely out of pain. If you try it and it causes pain, stop and wait a week or two before trying it again.

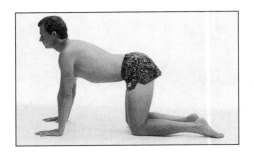

- To do the Back Builder, start on all fours, with your body in the shape of a table—arms and thighs straight down. You should be looking straight ahead.

- Find a spot on the wall or, if you are outside, on a distant fixed spot.

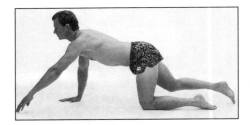

- Taking a breath in, extend your left arm out and your right leg back, "dragging" them along the floor.

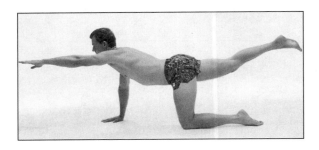

- As you exhale, raise your arm to shoulder level and your leg to waist level. Hold as you take in and let out two breaths.

- Inhale as you bring the legs down to the floor; exhale as you resume the starting pose.

- Taking a breath in, repeat the exercise with your right arm out and your left leg back. Repeat three times to each side.

Abdominal Crunches

Think of your abdomen as the front of your back. Again, since your low back is curved forward, extra weight in the belly tends to drag your spine forward and down, jamming joints. Strong abdominal muscles help keep this from happening.

This exercise gets its name from the way it crunches together your "abs."

- Start by lying on the floor, knees bent, feet flat on the floor.

- Clasp your hands together at the back of your head. Relax your shoulders.

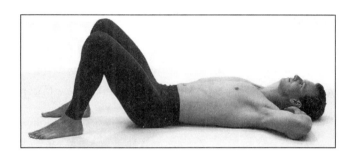

- Take a breath and, as you exhale, raise your torso up off the floor far enough that your shoulder blades just lift off the floor.

- Inhale and resume the starting position.

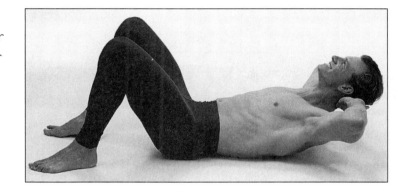

You might find it easier to do crunches if you imagine a large red arrow suspended above your belly, pointing straight down toward your belly button. As you breathe out, imagine the arrow pressing into your abdomen, and let this imaginary force raise you up. Also, it's important not to tuck your chin or strain your neck as you do your crunches. To keep your head and neck in the proper position, imagine an apple tucked under your chin, and don't let your jaw crush this apple as you raise yourself off the floor. Also, keep your arms relaxed, with your elbows dropped down toward the floor. It's natural to want to pull your elbows up toward your knees. Avoid this; let them stay out to the sides. Start with five stomach crunches and work your way up to twenty-five and then fifty each day.

The Pelvic Power Routine
Approximate workout time: 10 minutes

The following exercises should be done with an easy, rolling, rhythmic movement. They work very well when combined with the "Dynamic Relaxer" in chapter 8.

The Sacral Sit-Back

The flow of CSF around your spinal cord and brain is activated when you breathe. Normally, as we inhale, our tailbones move slightly forward, toward the front of our bodies, moving back as we exhale. We can increase the function of our CSF pump with this exercise.

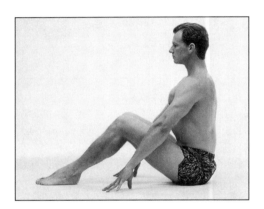

- Begin by sitting on the floor, knees bent, feet flat on the floor, arms outstretched and resting beside your thighs so that your fingers touch loosely on the floor. Your chin should be parallel to the floor. It's best to pick a spot on the wall in front of you and look at it while performing the Sacral Sit-Back.

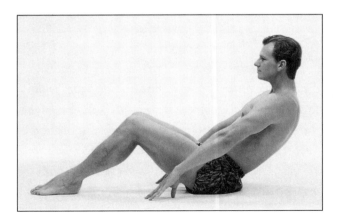

- As you inhale, move your upper body backward, dragging the fingers lightly over the floor, so that your chin moves back over your hips and your upper body forms roughly a forty-five-degree angle with the floor.

- Hold this position for a second or two and then breathe out, assuming the starting position. Repeat three times.

The Roundhouse

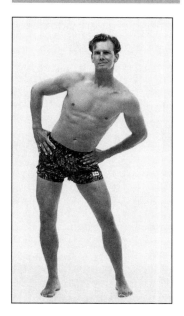 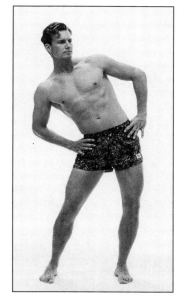 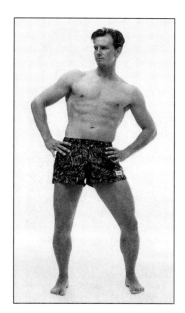

- Stand with your legs a bit more than shoulder-width apart, with your knees bent. You'll be doing a Hula-Hoop–type movement.

- Start by rotating your hips to the right, then backward, then left, then forward, making a circle with your hips. Get a nice, steady rhythm going.

- Do this exercise slowly but vigorously, pushing your hips out as far as is comfortable. If you experience pain, decrease your movement until the motion is comfortable.

- Circle ten times to the right, then switch directions, circling ten times to the left.

This exercise is particularly good for people suffering from minor hip pain. Also, you may notice an increased sexual desire after practicing the Roundhouse and the Pump for a few weeks.

The Pump

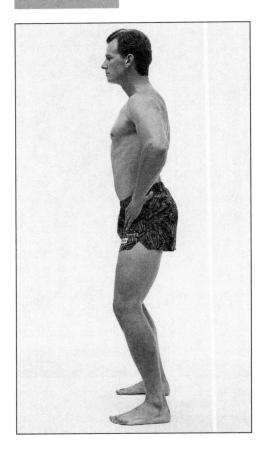

■ Stand with your feet shoulder-width apart. Begin by gently rocking your pelvis backward then forward with small, easy movements.

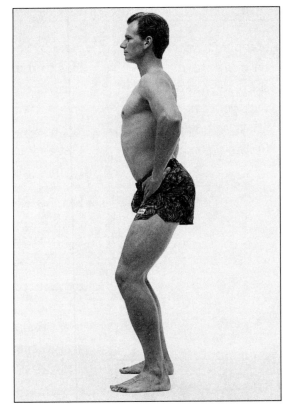

■ While breathing slowly and steadily, increase the movement of your pelvis until you're "swinging" it back and forth. Don't force the movements. Keep your knees bent.

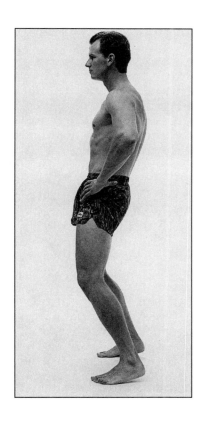

■ As you swing, your legs may begin to shake. Try to relax your pelvis and let this shaking sensation move its way up from your legs into your buttocks, belly, and back. Stop if you feel any discomfort.

■ Continue for twenty to thirty seconds or until the strain in your legs becomes uncomfortable. Try to increase your time spent "pumping" to one minute.

My Chiropractor's Advice:

7

HIGH VOLTAGE

[boosting your nervous system's power supply]

It's Thanksgiving. You've lasted through turkey, mashed potatoes, gravy, cranberry sauce, pumpkin pie, and a half dozen other diet terrorists. Your stomach feels like a beach-ball-size water balloon. Notice how drowsy you are, even before you start to wash the dishes?

You're tense. Your neck is so stiff you could use it to break boards. Admit it, wouldn't eating a piece of chocolate the size of a cat make you feel better?

The examples above demonstrate how the food we eat affects our nervous systems on every level, from the quality of our thoughts and emotions to how well we move.

An extreme example of this can be found in so-called hyperactive children, often labeled "out of control" by their parents and teachers. These kids have nervous systems firing at warp speed. Their attention is scattered; they often leap from one activity to another. Many are dosed with drugs to slow them down. More than 70 percent of such children, however, can be helped with a diet restricted in sugar, dyes, preservatives, and certain foods.

Shawn is a ten-year-old patient in our office, labeled hyperactive at six. "It was like raising a wild animal," said his mother, Beth.

At first Shawn's parents accepted their doctor's advice and put him on a commonly prescribed drug. "But we didn't like the idea of having him on drugs," said Beth. "We'd heard of the side effects, such as stunted growth and the delayed onset of puberty. So we went all-natural. We took him off the drugs, limited his diet, and structured his time better. Now he's a normal kid, and he knows that if he eats candy or drinks soda he loses control, so he stays away from them."

Incidentally, Beth has noticed even more improvement in Shawn's behavior under chiropractic care in our office. An examination showed that the first two bones in his neck were misaligned, putting pressure on nerves in the area. As we relieved nerve pressure in his body, it became easier for him to relax. "He's calmer and more focused. I think chiropractic has reduced the stress in him and helped him stay calm," says his mother.

QUANTITIES LIMITED

Why boost your nervous system's power supply through diet? It comes down to energy. A simple equation sums up why energy is so important:

$$\text{DECREASED STRESS} + \text{INCREASED ENERGY} = \text{MORE LIFE}$$

Decreasing stress in your life can help prevent blocks from forming and free energy currently trapped throughout your body.

Increasing energy means using food to give yourself a constant, internal source of power your nervous system can use to keep you healthy. We've seen how an overload of physical, emotional, mental, or chemical stress prevents us from functioning at top efficiency by blocking the flow of nerve impulses. By freeing energy trapped within you and increasing the energy you get from food, you increase your ability to build a better life. It's like setting free bottled lightning.

Our energy is limited. Like a pie, we can slice it in countless ways, but using it in one area of our lives means losing it in others. The good news is that you can bake a bigger pie by eating in a new way.

With a properly fueled nervous system, you'll have the energy after dinner to do something—anything—besides slump in front of the television; you'll work as effectively in the afternoon as in the morning. Maybe your love life will improve! Just as important, you'll increase your ability to withstand life's stresses.

I see this every day in practice. When people with abundant energy experience a stress such as a fall down a flight of stairs, a divorce, or challenges at work, they handle them with relative ease.

Not so with "couch potatoes." With as much energy as dead flashlights, they can't respond to crises. It's as if their energy reservoirs have been drought-stricken; they quickly dry up under pressure, and the person falls sick. The other day a new patient summed it up perfectly: "I don't have the energy to hold my body together anymore," she said at the end of a long day.

Another important aspect of the decreased-stress/increased-energy/more-life equation is that you need to decrease stress in order for your body to handle increased energy. If your nervous system is overloaded, with blocked areas inhibiting nerve flow, increasing the energy in your body can create feelings of anxiety, because the energy has nowhere to flow.

This is one reason why diets fail. If dieters start eating good, nutritious food, their energy rises. But the power influx runs into the same blocks already in their systems, creating anxiety.

I often witnessed this in the South when practicing in an area where black-eyed peas come cooked in fatback (raw fat from butchered pigs). In order to review their eating habits, I asked my patients to keep diet diaries in which they wrote down everything they ate and drank for an entire week.

Many of these reports showed patients eating eggs and bacon every day for breakfast, with fast food and a soda for lunch, and a dinner of meat, vegetables, and a sweet dessert. I was amazed at the number of people drinking four and five cans of soda each day. Fried chicken, hamburgers, hot dogs, bologna sandwiches, cheese-flavored snacks, candy bars . . . the diaries were nutrition nightmares!

However, as we began aligning their spines, many of these patients found it easier to change their eating habits. Large areas of their bodies had been functioning at less than 100 percent. As their bodies began to work better, they could handle the increased energy a good diet provided.

FILLING YOUR ENERGY RESERVOIR

In this chapter you'll learn how to boost your nervous system's power supply by:

- Making your digestive system more efficient
- Getting the most energy from any food you eat
- Eating to maximize your "core energy"
- Using simple breathing techniques to create more energy from your food
- Speeding up or slowing down your nervous system using food, vitamins, and herbs

CLEAN STREAK

Think of food as a beautifully wrapped gift. Inside is a wonderful present. It's golden and shining and gives off a warm glow. The energy in wholesome food is like that—a hidden treasure waiting to be unearthed.

Unfortunately, many times the eatable packages we eat never get unwrapped. Energy is locked in food. To get it out, we need a digestive system functioning like a five-year-old on Christmas morning, ripping off wrappings to get to the good stuff inside.

Food starts being transformed into energy when you chew. As your teeth grind and mash, saliva lubricates food and starts breaking down starches (for example, those contained in pasta and potatoes).

Once swallowed, your meal slides into your stomach. There it's squeezed and mixed with chemicals to break it down further. Different foods pass through the stomach at different rates. For example, carbohydrates such as bread are digested quickly; proteins, including meat and beans, take longer; and fatty foods take the longest of all. Cold foods slow the stomach down, while hot foods speed it up. Drinks, on the other hand, usually flow through the stomach directly into the intestines. (To get something into your system fast, put it in a warm liquid.)

When food in the stomach is nearly liquid it's squirted into the small intestine, which is about twenty-two feet long in adults and has walls thicker than a car tire's rubber inner tube. As food enters the intestine, more breakdown chemicals are added to it and digestion really gets going. Particles of foods that once ranged from chocolate-covered cherries to charcoal-broiled zucchini get broken into a handful of basic chemicals. These chemicals are then transported through the intestinal walls into your bloodstream. After a journey of twelve to forty-eight hours or more through the stomach and small intestine, unabsorbed "food" travels into the colon, where water and salt are removed, leaving solid waste.

WASH DAYS

Many chiropractors, including myself, recognize that a healthy digestive tract is crucial if you want to wring maximum energy from food. The best way to tune up your "food tube" is with a brief diet that cleans your intestinal walls, rests your digestive system so it can repair itself, and washes your colon of accumulated wastes.

I've found the easiest routine is a one- to three-day fruit cleansing regimen given to me by Dr. Jim Winer, a chiropractor in Pittsburgh, Pennsylvania. Dr. Winer recommends that you gradually prepare your body for the cleansing routine by eliminating junk food, dairy products, and meat from your diet for a week. During this time, drink eight glasses of distilled water, available at your grocery store, each day.

Distilled water, which is produced by heating water until it evaporates and then condensing the vapor back into liquid, contains nearly zero chemicals and minerals. Because of its purity, as it goes through your system, distilled water tends to draw out unwanted toxins stored in your cells.

Note: If you suffer from low blood sugar, diabetes, or other diseases, consult your chiropractor or another health professional qualified in nutritional matters before making any dietary changes.

Once you've primed your digestive system for a week, if you're in good health, begin the fruit diet by eating only fresh, uncooked fruit and drinking only distilled water or fruit juice for one to three days. Good fruit choices are oranges, grapefruit, apples, pears, peaches, plums, and nectarines. Be sure to thoroughly scrub all the fruit you eat to rid it of pesticides and waxes.

You may be hungry during the cleansing diet. Drinking lots of liquids helps take the edge off these unpleasant feelings. You may also notice some uncomfortable side effects such as loose stools, cramping, bloating, and even headaches while your body cleans itself out. As pleasant as a stubbed toe, these symptoms are usually a sign that the cleansing is working; they normally subside within a day or two. If you become concerned about what's happening to your body while it's getting an internal wash, consult a health professional who feels comfortable counseling you on nutritional needs.

Be gentle with yourself when using any cleansing diet. If your willpower wilts before the full three days, that's okay, because any rest you give your digestive system has a positive impact.

In his excellent book, *Dr. Winer's Basic Nutrition Handbook* (available from The Pain Release Clinic, 1320 East Carson Street, Pittsburgh, PA 15203; 412-431-7246), the chiropractor cautions, "How you end the fruit diet will be as important as the diet itself." He notes that whenever you return from a diet restricted to fruit, juices, or water you need to eat easily digestible foods first, gradually adding meals that are more difficult to digest.

"For fruit diets, begin with fruits and gradually work up to vegetables, then starches, then proteins and oils," says Dr. Winer. "If you have restricted yourself to fresh fruits for three days, then the first or second meal of the fourth day may be raw vegetables, such as a salad. Depending on the length of your fruit diet, continue eating only fruits or vegetables for one to three meals. Then introduce some grains or other starchy foods. After a few more meals, you may resume proteins, and lastly oils and fats. So after a three-day fruit diet you will spend another one to three days before resuming a full diet."

ENERGY EATING ETIQUETTE

I recommend a three-day cleansing fruit diet every three months to keep your digestive system in top condition. In between, you can trap more energy from your food by becoming more aware of *how* you eat. The following eating practices will help extract maximum energy from your food, decrease stress on your digestive tract, and in the process clear up many common digestion problems such as excess gas and indigestion:

- **Eat less.** Stuffing yourself strains your system's ability to digest what you eat. Also, overeating drains energy. You may have noticed that after a large lunch or dinner, nothing is more appealing than a long nap. That's because after meals your nervous system diverts blood to the stomach and intestines from other areas of your body, including your brain. "We've seen it demonstrated time and again in laboratory experiments: As calorie intake per meal is increased, mental performance afterward drops sharply," notes Dr. Judith J. Wurtman, a researcher at the Massachusetts Institute of Technology and the author of *Managing Your Mind and Mood Through Food.*

I once taught industrial safety classes in which I would warn workers that a peak time for industrial accidents occurs after lunch, when workers' stomachs are full and their brains "empty."

- **Eat in a peaceful atmosphere.** As Deepak Chopra writes in his best-selling book *Perfect Health*: "Your body is tremendously alert while you are eating. Your stomach cells are aware of the conversation at the dinner table, and if they hear harsh words, the stomach will know the distress."
- **Eat in a comfortable position.** Consuming food while you're standing, walking, or driving leads to indigestion, because you're not concentrating on eating.
- **Eat only when you're hungry.** Sure, eating chocolate might feel good when you're tense, but it's a sure way to put on pounds and produce belching and intestinal gas.
- **Avoid ice-cold or very hot food and drink.** These will alter your stomach's normal actions.
- **Chew your food slowly and thoroughly.** Digestion starts in the mouth, so get it off to a good start by turning your food to mush before you swallow.
- **Limit how much you drink with your food.** Drinking a lot of water or other beverages with your food dilutes the juices your stomach produces to digest your food.
- **Bless your food.** Studies show that an "attitude of gratitude" when it comes to the food we eat helps us digest it better.

BUILDING CORE ENERGY

Since becoming a chiropractor, I've grown to realize there are five key components to good health: one-hundred-percent nerve flow leading to one-hundred-percent function; a good mental attitude; enough rest; proper nutrition; and sufficient exercise. Of the five keys, none is more important than good, basic nutrition. It's what and how you eat day in and out that determines the amount of your energy, what I term "core energy."

I'm not a diet guru, and I don't think you need one, because the greatest nutritionist in the world is already inside you, turning everything from sandwiches to spumoni into energy every day. What we all need is a good plan for working with this intelligence inside us.

YOU'VE GOT THE RHYTHM

You can make it easy for your body to create energy from what you eat. All you need to do is work with the natural cycles within you for taking in, breaking down, and eliminating food. These cycles are as follows:

- **Roughly noon to 8:00 P.M.:** Time for eating and digestion.
- **8:00 P.M. to 4:00 A.M.:** The time when you should be absorbing the chemicals from the food you've digested, using them to repair your body from the inside out and storing energy for the next day.
- **4:00 A.M. to noon:** The time when you should be eliminating wastes.

Since your body should be eliminating food in the morning, it's best to eat something that's easily digested for breakfast. That way your body isn't working to digest a heavy meal while at the same time trying to eliminate yesterday's waste. Fresh fruit is the best choice. Loaded with good things your body needs to stay healthy, it's also the most easily digested food. Eating bananas, melons, peaches, nectarines, or grapefruit for breakfast won't slow you down. These are also good sources of fiber, helping to keep your food tube clean and fresh.

It's best not to eat other foods with fruit. I tell patients to wait at least a half hour after eating fruit to eat something else. If you can stick with fruit until lunch, all the better. Eating a midmorning fruit snack helps keep your energy high.

Another good way to respect your body's natural cycles is to eat your last meal early in the evening. Try to not eat anything after 8:00 P.M. In today's world it's often difficult, but if you can finish dinner by 6:00 P.M., your body will be able to rest better at night. You'll also sleep better if you avoid meat, dairy products, and other proteins at dinner. These are hard to digest, and make your body work overtime when it should be resting.

WATER WORLD

Your body is 70 percent water, so it's always made sense to me that most of the food we eat should also be 70 percent water. That's why I tell my patients to eat a grocery bag full of fruits and vegetables each week. Only about 30 percent of what you eat should be concentrated, low-water foods like meat, bread, grains, and dairy products. While these foods provide essential nutrients, eating too much of them saps us of energy because they are much harder to digest.

This philosophy conforms to today's emphasis on low-fat diets. Most fruits and vegetables contain very little or no fat. The best way to lose weight is to substitute fruits and vegetables for high-fat foods, while exercising regularly. If you adopt such a lifestyle, you'll slim down with ease.

COMBO MEALS

One of the best ways to work with your body is to avoid combining foods that confuse your stomach. For example, meat requires your stomach to produce acidic digestive juices, while potatoes are digested with the chemical opposite, alkaline juices. Vegetables are "neutral" and can be digested by either secretion.

Because your body is intelligent, when you swallow a piece of steak, your stomach automatically produces the right chemicals to break it down. But if you eat steak and potatoes, two opposite chemicals are produced, neutralizing each other. This leaves undigested food in the stomach far longer than necessary, consuming energy you could use for other purposes.

The best way to avoid this energy drain is to eat only one type of concentrated food at a time. Some "bad" but common combinations are listed in *Fit for Life,* by Harvey and Marilyn Diamond, a great book giving a complete explanation of the benefits of proper food combining. Off-limits combos include meat and potatoes, fish and rice, chicken and noodles, eggs and toast, cheese and bread, and cereal and milk.

The best food combinations are meat, potatoes, or pasta with vegetables and a salad, or a salad with cheese.

As you might guess, food combining is the most difficult part of eating for maximum energy—it's hard to eat a hamburger on a bed of lettuce rather than a bun. Pizza is technically off limits, though many people would choose bamboo slivers under their fingernails rather than give up a spicy slice of their favorite pie. Try eating only fruit for breakfast. You'll be properly combining food one third of the time. Then try to steer clear of improper food combinations at lunch and dinner whenever possible.

MEATY ISSUES

While fat takes the longest to leave your stomach, protein takes more total digestion time than any other food. Eating a lot of protein, particularly meat and dairy products, puts wear and tear on your food tube like nothing else. Try to limit protein intake to one serving each day. A good portion is about the size of a single chicken breast.

POWER SURGES

Sometimes you'd like your nervous system to relax and unwind. At other times you'd like it to function faster than a lawyer writing out his bill. You can accomplish either of these goals by eating the right food. In fact, by choosing to eat certain foods you can adapt your nervous system to any situation. The key is to feed your brain in the right way.

Your brain manufactures chemicals from what you eat. It produces two "alertness chemicals" and one that tends to calm you. To get your brain functioning faster, eat foods creating an abundance of alertness chemicals in your brain. To calm down, take in meals increasing calm chemical levels. Here's how to do it:

In *Managing Your Mind and Mood Through Food,* Dr. Wurtman says you can energize your brain by eating protein foods containing as little fat and/or carbohydrate as possible. These include fish, skinless chicken, veal,

125

and lean beef trimmed of all visible fat. Also good are nonfat cottage cheese, skimmed or nonfat milk, nonfat yogurt, dried peas and beans, lentils, and tofu and other soybean-based foods.

You can eat other foods along with your protein. For example, green leafy vegetables are "neutral" as they affect the brain, so eating to boost brainpower doesn't have to mean improper food combining. For example, at lunch you might eat fish and vegetables. If you do mix proteins and carbohydrates, you need to eat the protein first, thereby blocking the effects of carbohydrates consumed at the same meal.

Let's say you're facing a particularly tough mental challenge, from spending hours planning the family budget to putting together an important project at work. You've got to be "on." What foods to eat?

Breakfast is the meal that least affects brainpower. Apparently our natural bodily rhythms and the absorption of nutrients from the previous day energize us in the morning. If we stay away from high-fat foods at breakfast, we'll be relatively alert. A good morning wake-up routine, fresh fruit, and a glass of fruit juice will get your brain cells shouting at each other. If you need a snack before lunch, try more fresh fruit or plain, nonfat yogurt.

To keep your brain cooking at lunch, try tuna mixed with celery and moistened with lemon juice and olive oil, along with a salad and nonfat dressing, or broiled chicken breast, again with salad or vegetables.

Want your thinking machine to steamroll into the night? Then eat broiled fish or chicken, again with salad and vegetables.

JET FUEL

Of course, drinks and foods containing the drug caffeine (that's right, caffeine isn't only a drug, but a powerful one at that) improve mental performance.

"Caffeine is a mind-accelerating mood booster," says Dr. Wurtman. She reports that in studies at MIT, caffeine increased the reaction times, accuracy, and concentration of test subjects.

Caffeine also improves physical performance. In Tibet, where elevations average fourteen thousand feet and most tourists can hike about ten of them before breaking into a pant, tea aids endurance. Locals figure the distance between villages by the tea needed to trek the journey, with three cups equaling about eight kilometers.

In chapter 4 we saw how using caffeine puts you on an energy roller coaster. You'll need to decide whether its positive effects on mental and physical performance are worth jeopardizing your overall health. Like all drugs, if you are going to use caffeine, you should do so only when absolutely necessary.

LOUNGE ACT

Now let's say you want to calm down. Foods that slow your nervous system include bread, crackers, muffins, pasta, potatoes, rice, corn, oatmeal, candy, cookies, pie, cake, ice cream, jams, jellies, syrup, and honey.

So, after amazing yourself all day with your lightninglike mental prowess, for dinner you might enjoy spaghetti with meatless marinara sauce, a salad, vegetables like broccoli or asparagus, and Italian bread. A half hour before bedtime, snack on toast with margarine, oatmeal, or fig bars, along with a relaxing tea (see below).

BREATH FRESHENERS

One reason many people experience a continual energy crisis isn't for lack of good food, but the absence of a crucial ingredient your body uses to turn food into fuel: air. More specifically, the oxygen in air, which is used to "burn" the chemicals obtained from food breakdown. You can eat all you want, but without oxygen your energy will dry up.

Most of us breathe halfway into our chests, but to energize ourselves we need to pack air into the lungs. If you're like me (and 99 percent of the other people in the Western Hemisphere), you won't be able to breathe for energy all the time. It takes conscious attention, and we're usually concentrating on something else. The trick is to use the exercises described below whenever you have some spare time. For example, incorporate them into your morning wake-up routine. Do them when you commute to work or when you go to the bathroom. Breathe for energy before you exercise or eat. Build them into your schedule so you're breathing for energy at least once a day, more often if possible. Combined with eating well, the next three exercises will catapult your core energy to new heights.

Breathing for Energy Routine
Approximate workout time: 5 minutes

Belly Breathing

This may be the most powerful high-energy breathing technique known to man. It fills the lungs with air and increases the oxygen available to your bloodstream.

■ To belly-breathe: Sit or stand in a comfortable position. Place a hand on your belly, just under the navel. As you inhale through your nose, imagine your belly is a big balloon you're filling with air. Fill the balloon with your breath, feeling your hand getting pushed forward. Keep breathing in. Fill the middle of your chest, imagining the balloon getting bigger. Imagine it starting to expand into the space in front of you, touching the walls and rising toward the ceiling. Keep inhaling, and feel the top of your chest expand.

■ When you've filled your entire chest, hold the breath for a slow count of four, then begin exhaling through your nose.

■ As you breathe out, gently push in your belly with your hand, exhaling the air at the bottom of your lungs first, then pushing the air out of the middle and top of your chest. Repeat slowly four times.

The 1-4-2 Breath

This is another technique for getting more oxygen into your lungs.

■ Start by slowly breathing in to the count of four ("one-thousand one, one-thousand two," and so on). Next, hold the breath four times as long, to a count of sixteen. Afterward, breathe out, expelling all the air, to a count of eight.

■ Repeat four times.

■ You can increase the times for inhaling, holding, and exhaling the breath, but keep the 1-4-2 ratio. For example, inhale to a count of eight, hold for a count of thirty-two, and exhale for a count of sixteen.

This is an excellent exercise to do while driving to work, leaving you fresh and clearheaded.

The Sixty-Second Exhaler

When we inhale we energize our bodies; when we exhale we naturally relax. This accounts for the good feeling we get after a long sigh. By exaggerating the exhalation part of our breath, we relax and "reset" our normal breath pattern for deeper breathing.

■ Using Belly Breathing, fill your chest with air. Now clamp your teeth together and press your tongue against your upper teeth, exhaling so that you produce a hissing sound.

■ On your first attempts, you may only be able to hiss for fifteen to twenty seconds, but with practice you'll be able to increase that time. Your goal is to push the air out of your lungs in a long, extended hiss lasting sixty seconds.

A Good Night's Sleep

No single formula guarantees everyone a good night's sleep, but here are some tips on finding the best way for you to rest:

1. We spend nearly a third of our lives in bed, so it pays to invest in a quality mattress. Most mattresses need to be replaced every five to eight years, no matter what their warranties. Less expensive mattresses won't last that long. Plan on spending from three hundred to five hundred dollars for a quality mattress and box spring.

In general, most people do better on the firmest mattress that's comfortable. I've found most patients with back and neck problems do not do as well sleeping on a water bed.

2. A quality pillow is a must. Most people do best on those with a dished-out center section. This shape allows your neck to rest in alignment with the rest of the spine. Plan on spending at least twenty dollars for a quality pillow.

3. The best sleeping positions are on your back, with a small pillow tucked under your knees, or on your side, with a small pillow tucked between your knees. These positions help keep your spine properly aligned throughout the night.

HIGH-TEST ADDITIVES

Food and air are the basic building blocks of core energy. However, some vitamins and herbs help build a physically stronger nervous system and can be used to speed up or slow down how fast it works.

Vitamins for Nervous System Health

Some vitamins protect the brain, spinal cord, and nerves from attack by "free radicals." In his book *Antioxidant Revolution,* Dr. Kenneth H. Cooper describes free radicals as

> *unstable oxygen molecules darting crazily about and crashing into other particles and tissues. Chemical studies have demonstrated that the impact of those particles actually produces bursts of light. Their movement and appearance are volatile and unpredictable in comparison with other molecules because they have one or more unpaired electrons in their outer orbits. That deficiency in their structure causes them to seek out other molecules with which they can combine.*

Free radicals damage cells within us by weakening their sacklike walls. It's as if each one of the trillions of cells making up our bodies were encased in a plastic sandwich bag. Free radicals poke holes in the bag, crippling the cells so they start acting old and worn out.

Some scientists believe free radicals are one reason many people's brains deteriorate with time. The reason is that our brains contain a high proportion of unsaturated fat, a favorite food of free radicals.

Other vitamins help nervous system cells "eat." For example, the only "food" used by brain cells is glucose, a sugar carried in blood. Vitamins that help nerve cells to use glucose increase brain function.

The vitamins your nervous system craves are listed below:

BETA-CAROTENE

Beta-carotene is a fat-soluble antioxidant used by the body to make vitamin A. Your best source of beta-carotene is several servings of fruits and vegetables each day. Particularly good are dark green vegetables, fruits, carrots, sweet potatoes, tomatoes, spinach, squash, cantaloupe, mango, papaya, apricots, and broccoli. If you use supplements, take 25,000 International Units (IUs) or about 15 milligrams (mg) per day.

VITAMIN B COMPLEX

Including a B-complex supplement in your daily diet is like hiring a personal trainer for your nerves. Vitamins B_1 and B_{12} help transform glucose into energy. B_3 improves the ability of red blood cells to carry oxygen to your brain. B_5 and B_6 are used to make chemicals that carry messages between brain cells. A good natural source of vitamin B complex is wholewheat bread. If you take supplements, look for those containing a minimum of 100 milligrams (mg) of B_1, B_2, B_6, niacin, pantothenic acid, and choline, and 100 micrograms (mcg) of B_{12}, folic acid, and biotin.

VITAMIN C

The body's chief antioxidant, Vitamin C is concentrated around the brain and spinal cord to fight off free radicals. Good sources for vitamin C include citrus fruits, cantaloupe, broccoli, brussels sprouts, cauliflower, carrots, and tomatoes. Vitamin C is so important that I recommend that patients use supplements to make sure they're getting enough. Since your body doesn't store Vitamin C, it's important to take it in the morning and again sometime in the late afternoon. I like to take a chewable 500 mg vitamin C tablet after breakfast and again sometime before dinner.

VITAMIN E

Again, a great antioxidant, vitamin E helps keep your brain youthful and vigorous. Natural sources include corn and sunflower oil, almonds, hazelnuts, eggs, and butter. If you use supplements, take 400 IUs or 400 mg in capsule form daily.

Customizing Nervous System Function with Nerve Herbs

Some herbs are antioxidants, others increase blood flow to your brain, and still others speed up or slow down nervous system function. Those thought to have the greatest impact on your body's master control system include the following:

GINKGO BILOBA

More than $500 million worth of ginkgo is sold each year in Europe. The reason for the rage is that ginkgo improves blood flow to the brain and helps it use glucose. It's been dubbed an anti-aging substance because it seems to reverse some of the most common "getting older but not better" symptoms, such as decreased memory and impotence. Recommended dosage is one 80 mg capsule twice each day.

GINSENG

Ginseng benefits the brain because it's a so-called adaptogen, a substance increasing the body's resistance to stress and normalizing its functions. Numerous studies document ginseng's ability to improve concentration, memory, and learning. Quality counts when buying this herb. Most cheap products don't deliver benefits because of the special requirements needed to handle ginseng. Look for a product made with whole, unprocessed, six-year-old Chinese roots (ask your health-food store or herb dealer for details). Take one 50 mg capsule per day.

VALERIAN

Recommended by herbalists for anxiety and insomnia, valerian is a wonderful nervous system relaxant. In West Germany it's an active ingredient in about one hundred over-the-counter tranquilizers and sleep aids. Valerian is available as an extract or as a powder, in capsules. The extract has a strong, sweet odor, but if you can get past the smell, it works well in tea preparations. As a sleep aid, take one half to one teaspoon of the extract, or two 150 mg capsules, a half hour before bed. As a daytime relaxant, take one 150 mg capsule with breakfast, lunch, and dinner. Note: some people react strongly to this herb, and shouldn't drive or do work requiring intense concentration after taking it; take one 150 mg capsule on a morning when you'll be home to test your reaction.

CHAMOMILE

Another proven nervous system quieter. Unlike valerian, chamomile extract has a nice smell and can be added to herbal teas, which can be drunk throughout a stress-filled day. Plenty of chamomile teas are also available. As a sleep aid, drink a cup of chamomile tea before bed or use one half to one teaspoon of the extract in your favorite herbal tea about a half hour before bed. As a daytime relaxant, take one 75 mg tablet or capsule with breakfast, lunch, and dinner.

Bringing Herbs Home

Good herb stores can be harder to find than fun-loving bankers. Not to worry. The following companies offer free catalogs showcasing fields of herbal products:

- The Vitamin Trader
  6501 Fourth Street, NW
  Albuquerque, NM 87107-5800
  1-800-334-9310

- HerbPharm's Whole Herb Catalog
  P.O. Box 116
  Williams, OR 97544
  1-800-348-4372

AN ENERGY EATER'S GUIDE

How do you integrate all the strategies previously outlined for controlling nervous system function through diet and supplementation? Eating to create a large supply of core energy, along with the sensible supplementation of your diet with the vitamins and herbs mentioned above, should bake you a big enough energy pie to launch you through 90 percent of your days.

However, sometimes you may want to really crank up the brainpower, and at other times turn down your nervous system's volume control. On the next two pages you'll find two sample menus, one for maximizing nervous system function, another for those days when you want to relax.

Please note: The Blast-Your-Brain-Out-of-Befuddlement Menu is low in calories and fat, because your brain works better when your body is slightly hungry. On the special days when you use this diet, maintain a comfortable feeling of fullness by drinking plenty of liquids, snacking on fruit, and eating extra-large portions of vegetables, if needed.

The Blast-Your-Brain-out-of-Befuddlement Menu

Breakfast

fresh fruit (bananas, strawberries, melon, etc.)

or

a fresh fruit "smoothie." To make this morning health booster, in a blender combine 1 cup ice with 2 bananas and six strawberries (you don't need the ice if you use frozen strawberries) and 1 cup orange juice. Blend until smooth.

and

fruit juice

or

decaffeinated coffee or tea

Supplement this with:

ginkgo biloba
ginseng
vitamin C
B complex vitamins
vitamin E

and

four repetitions of the 1-4-2 Breath, Belly Breathing, or the Sixty-Second Exhaler

Lunch

1 can water-packed tuna mixed with chopped celery and scallions, moistened with olive oil/lemon dressing

or

1 serving of broiled skinless chicken or fish

or

1 tofu burger, served without a bun on a bed of lettuce and tomato

and

1 serving of fresh vegetables, stir-fried or steamed

and

salad with nonfat dressing

and

decaffeinated coffee or tea if desired

Supplement this with:

four repetitions of the 1-4-2 Breath, Belly Breathing, or the Sixty-Second Exhaler

Dinner

| | Supplement this with: |

1 serving broiled skinless chicken or fish

or

1 tofu burger on a bed of lettuce and tomato

and

vegetables and salad

and

decaffeinated coffee or tea if needed

vitamin C

and

four repetitions of the 1-4-2 Breath, Belly Breathing, or the Sixty-Second Exhaler

The Make-My-Mind-a-Soft-Soufflé Menu

Breakfast

Supplement this with:

fresh fruit or a fresh fruit smoothie

and/or

toast with jelly or jam, or **bagel,** if a smoothie doesn't satisfy your hunger

and

chamomile tea

vitamins C and E

B complex vitamin

valerian in capsule form

and

four repetitions of the Sixty-Second Exhaler

Lunch

Supplement this with:

vegetarian chili

and

fresh vegetables, steamed or stir-fried

and

salad with nonfat dressing

and

bread with butter

and

fruit

and

chamomile tea

valerian in capsule form

and

four repetitions of the Sixty-Second Exhaler

Dinner

pasta with meatless marinara sauce

or

mashed potatoes and nonfat gravy

and

fresh vegetables

and

salad

and

bread with butter

and

chamomile tea

fruit dessert

with a bedtime snack of

bowl of oatmeal

or

2 fig bars

and

chamomile tea with one teaspoon valerian root extract

Supplement this with:

valerian in capsule form

and

four repetitions of the Sixty-Second Exhaler

My Chiropractor's Advice:

8

BLOCK BUSTER EXERCISE

[the new neuromuscular health]

Trish kicked her right leg high in the air as the music pounded and the instructor yelled, "Do it again! Harder! Harder! Right leg down, left leg up! Right leg up, left arm out!"

Another ten minutes of pulse-pounding kicks, twists, and lunges, and the aerobics class was over. Sweat dripped from Trish's back as if from a faucet. The air was thick with overheated lungs pouring perspiration into the room. Trish was drained, and it felt good. Her ears still ringing from the amplified workout, she thought about how tense her muscles had been just an hour before, and wondered, "Why can't my body always feel this good?"

As Bill flew off the ski jump traveling at highway speed, he knew something was dreadfully wrong. Way off the smooth arc he normally rode through the air, a crosswind twisted him to the left. The ground was twenty-five yards away and closing fast. He tried to correct his balance, but there wasn't enough time. As he hit the snow, his body seemed to come apart at the seams. He tumbled in a split-legged, sprawling mass down the ski run, tearing muscles and ligaments in his neck and back. Six months after his accident and more than two hundred hours of strengthening/stretching rehabilitation exercises behind him, Bill was ready to jump again. His body felt strong, flexible, and agile, his muscles ready to react to any demands made of them.

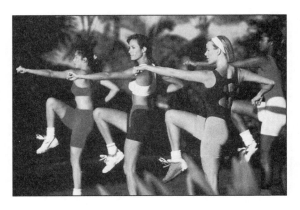

As he stood in the starting gate, however, his heart began pounding. Uncontrollable panic gripped him. He began to shake. Fear had taken up residence in the muscles of his chest, arms, and legs.

In step. Aerobic training sends increased oxygen and nutrients throughout your body.

Trish and Bill illustrate the power of exercise to transform our bodies. They also demonstrate that vigorous workouts alone will not provide you with the total health you seek.

MOVING VIOLATIONS

Hundreds of studies have demonstrated the value of regular exercise. "Use it or lose it" sums up why exercise is crucial if you want to live in a healthy, vibrant body. If we use them, our bodies respond by working better.

For example, if we take regular aerobics classes our hearts, lungs, arteries, capillaries, and veins become really good at pumping blood. The benefits are astounding. Fresh blood delivers vital oxygen and nutrients to our cells while clearing out cellular waste.

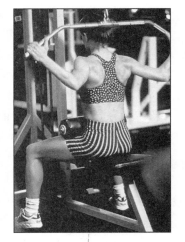

Weight training provides different but similarly sound benefits. Greater muscle mass burns calories faster, so a person who lifts weights and builds muscle can eat more while maintaining his or her shape. Muscle mass also has a great deal to do with physical stamina, our overall vigor, and our ability to fight fatigue.

Bulk packaging. Weight training's benefits go far beyond thinner thighs.

Not surprisingly, many of the benefits of exercise result from its positive effects on our nervous systems. You may have heard of endorphins. These are painkilling, mood-elevating chemicals manufactured by the brain during exercise. They circulate in the blood, providing a natural "high."

Your brain also thinks differently during exercise. It's been shown that you start thinking in a more relaxed manner twenty minutes into a thirty-minute run, and keep thinking this way after the exercise is over.

Exercise boosts our well-being, too. Studies show running to be at least as effective as psychotherapy in alleviating moderate depression. In addition, our self-concept, short-term memory, and intellectual functioning are all helped by training our bodies to work better.

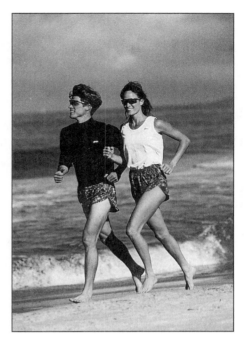

Un-conscious. Exercise helps our minds relax and unwind.

YOU SAY YOU WANT AN EVOLUTION

Most of us have experienced some of the benefits that exercise provides our brains and bodies, but few have considered how exercise can help the two work together.

That's changing. During the Charles Atlas era and up until Arnold Schwarzenegger was winning his Mr. Universe titles, health and fitness were associated with large, well-defined muscles. In the 1970s that changed, as the emphasis shifted to getting our hearts and lungs in shape through aerobic exercises like running. In the 1980s, cross-training developed, as the concept of achieving a balance between big muscles and strong cardiovascular systems took center stage.

Perhaps because we live in a "stressed for success" society, today a fourth dimension is being added to the shape of shaping up, as the link between mind, body, and exercise becomes more clearly understood. As one women's magazine puts it: "Mindless repetitions are out. What's in: exercising your brain as well as your body."

What's emerging is a new field, neuromuscular health, referring to how our brains interact with our muscles to influence our well-being. The goal of neuromuscular health is to eliminate blocks to the flow of nerve energy so that our nervous systems can control and coordinate every function of our bodies with effectiveness and ease.

MOVING VIOLATIONS

The problem with conventional exercise is that while it drains tension from our systems, it often doesn't get rid of blocks in our bodies. As discussed in chapter 3, blocks are areas within us where nervous system overload has created pinched nerves and/or tight muscles and joints, areas that are inflexible, where nerve impulses become trapped or distorted, where life doesn't flow. That's why Trish's body feels great after an aerobics class, but she wonders why that feeling quickly fades and she's again filled with tension. It's why Bill could spend months strengthening and stretching his muscles, only to have them betray him at the moment of truth.

It often feels as though muscles have minds of their own. When our shoulders tense, it seems like something *inside* the muscle is tightening up, causing us to become locked up or blocked in that part of our body. *But blocks don't originate in muscles. They are rooted in our brains.*

Although it feels as if individual muscles contract and relax on their own, the overall action of the more than two hundred muscles in your body is controlled by your brain. To achieve neuromuscular health, you need to change the nerve connections between your brain and body.

BUILDING BLOCKS

If you watch babies move, you'll notice they lack coordination. This is because the nerve connections between their brains and muscles aren't fully developed. This is part of being human. Many "lower" animals pop out of their shells, cocoons, or pouches with a whole set of preprogrammed reflexes that let them eat, crawl, swim, or fly within a short time; they don't need much experience to learn how to survive.

We lack many built-in reflexes, and have to learn virtually everything. This turns out not to be a drawback: our capacity to learn is what makes us the most adaptable creatures on the planet.

Our brains learn to control our muscles through trial and error. When a baby wants to crawl, its brain sends messages to its muscles saying, "Move!" Because there aren't many solid brain-muscle connections, the movements are haphazard. But the baby's brain uses receptors in the muscles and joints that tell it where its body's parts are and how they're moving. It detects any muscular efforts that aren't helping the baby move, and weeds them out. Bit by bit, the baby moves more efficiently. This is how brain/muscle connections form.

A more advanced example is learning to ride a bike. At first it's hard just to climb on. Then you keep falling off. After a while, however, your muscles get together with your brain and you learn to balance on the bike, eventually getting to the point where you hop on your bike and take off down the street as easily as drinking a glass of water.

This same process is repeated thousands of times as you mature. Over the years you develop thousands of patterns that control the interaction between your brain and muscles.

Some of these patterns aren't healthy. For example, let's say you break your right ankle. To prevent further injury, the brain automatically shifts your weight to the left leg, creating a limp. Say you limp for eight weeks. A muscular pattern is established. The brain keeps the muscles of the right hip contracted, creating a tilted pelvis and forming a block in your body. The contraction may remain long after the ankle heals. In fact, it can stay until the day you die, unless the mind-muscle connection is somehow "reprogrammed."

Surgery can also form blocks. Gerry came to our clinic suffering from right-shoulder pain. During our consultation she related that her pain had first appeared eight months after she underwent a mastectomy of the right breast. On examination, I found that the muscles attaching her chest to her shoulder were extremely tight. The surgery had caused these muscles to "cringe" in a protective reflex that lasted long after her surgical scars had healed.

Strong emotions also imprint the mind-muscle connection. For example, if you're walking across the street and suddenly hear a loud horn blast nearby, your muscles immediately tighten in a startle response: within fourteen milliseconds, your jaw muscles contract; twenty milliseconds later, your eyes clamp shut and your shoulders and neck muscles constrict, raising your shoulders and drawing your head forward; thirty milliseconds later, your elbows bend and your hands turn palms-down. Your abdominal muscles contract, bending you forward, pulling down your rib cage and restricting your breathing. Next your crotch muscles tighten and your toes lift up.

What happens to a five-year-old boy who is routinely beaten by his father? The startle response takes root in his muscles, even when his father isn't around.

As connections form between your body and brain, your life history becomes embedded in your muscles. An underlying pattern of muscular contractions is built up as you experience emotions, traumas, and different mental states.

Trish can wash away muscular tension with exercise. But in a short while her brain resumes control, resetting her muscle tone based on her history and emotional state. If she keeps doing aerobics, her body will keep changing, as new movement patterns join the countless others in her brain. Her neuromuscular health will improve, but she may never enjoy her level of post-workout relaxation unless she actively reprograms her muscles to rid her body of blocked areas.

SHOW STOPPERS

Your neuromuscular health affects your performance at every level. Can you see why it's so difficult to control your posture through conscious effort? If you concentrate, you can sit up straight and tall. But as soon as you think of something else, your brain subconsciously sets the tone of every muscle in your body, based on past neuromuscular programming. To change posture, you need to input new information into your brain.

Many people's chronic pains are caused by faulty neuromuscular health. Brenda worked at a sewing machine in a garment factory. Each day she sewed about fifty shirts, using the same motions of her back, shoulders, and arms in assembling each one. A fall from a roof as a teenager had left her with contracted muscles in her neck and shoulders, but she wasn't aware of it. After six months of sewing, she developed bursitis in both her shoulders, along with pain in her right wrist. A large part of Brenda's recovery involved realigning her spine in order to change the movement patterns in her neck and shoulders. This let her work in a more relaxed manner. In a matter of weeks the bursitis and hand pain cleared up, and she was able to sew sixty shirts a day without pain.

BRING BACK THAT FLOWING FEELING

Until now, we've focused on how your brain sets muscle tone throughout your body. But muscle tone affects brain function, too. For example, if the receptors in your abdominal muscles tell your brain that your belly is tight and tense, this information alters the chemicals manufactured in your brain that influence your moods and emotions. You may have noticed that when you're angry, your body tenses. When you relax, though, it's hard even to feel angry.

Tense muscles make for tense minds. Soft, flexible muscles lead to flexible, open attitudes. If we use exercise to stay physically relaxed, emotions that might otherwise overwhelm our nervous systems and lead to blocks in our bodies can instead make our lives more vibrant.

If you want one-hundred-percent nerve flow, you need to reprogram the connections between your mind and muscles, releasing patterns that make your body tight and tense. Described on the next several pages are two exercises that can help.

The Block Buster Exercise Routines
Approximate workout time: 5 to 10 minutes

The Neurological Flush

There are more muscle receptors in your neck than anywhere else in your body. They send information to your brain about your neck's position, and the brain uses this information to help set muscle tone throughout your body.

If the receptors send poor information to the brain, your brain will inappropriately tighten or loosen muscles. The Neurological Flush "resets" receptors in your neck so that your brain gets correct information on which to set muscle tone.

When Bill the skier developed a fear of ski jumps, he went to a chiropractor. The chiropractor went to work on Bill's brain by showing him how to do the Neurological Flush. After doing the exercise each day for several weeks, Bill was soaring again.

This exercise is especially good to do before playing sports, because it enhances balance, hand-eye coordination, and reaction time.

Before trying it, do the following test:

- Stand about eighteen inches away from a light switch. Hold your arms so that your elbows are bent and your hands are just in front of your shoulders, index fingers pointing up toward the ceiling.

- Look at the light switch and extend your right hand out so that your index finger touches the switch. Bring your arm back and do the same movement with your left hand.

- Now look at the light switch again, but this time close your eyes before trying to hit the switch with the tip of your right finger. Did you hit the switch? Try to hit the switch with your left hand. If you're like most people, you may miss the switch with either your right or left hand.

Now do the Neurological Flush:

- Sit or stand about six inches away from a wall, and prop a plastic ball or firm cushion behind your neck.

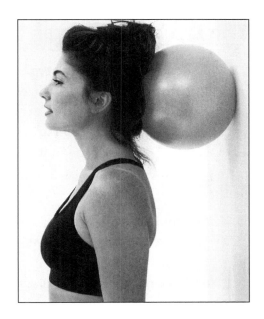

- With the back of your head resting on the ball, push your head back, as if you were trying to touch the wall with the back of your head. Repeat this motion fairly quickly thirty times, to the cadence "one-thousand one, one-thousand two," and so on. The muscle receptors in your neck will start sending new information to your brain.

- Try the light-switch test again and see if this new input helps you function better.

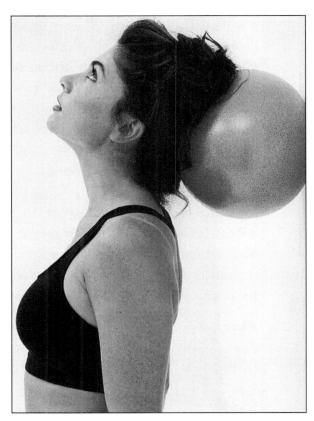

The Dynamic Relaxer

The drained feeling you get after a good workout is the result of your muscles releasing chronic tension. This exercise helps eliminate blocks in your body so that you can achieve that same feeling all the time.

In doing the Dynamic Relaxer you'll need to forget some of the activities you associate with exercise, such as sweating, grunting, and forcing your body beyond its usual limits. This exercise requires thinking *as well as* doing. *The following guidelines will help you get the most from it:*

- **Move slowly.** Moving slowly lets you notice tension in your body and gives you the chance to release it. Think about how, exactly, your body is moving as you practice each motion.
- **Make your movements small.** Unlike traditional exercises, in this routine you're gently exploring your body's limits, and then giving the body a chance to move beyond them.
- **Relax.** Using a lot of effort makes it hard for your brain to notice what changes it needs to make to improve your mind-muscle connections. Conventional exercise, with its reliance on muscular effort, force, and speed, actually restricts your brain's ability to work on your body's behalf.

  For example, if you've lifted a thirty-pound dumbbell and a fly lands on it, all the effort you're using to lift the dumbbell eliminates your ability to feel the fly's weight. If you hold a feather and a fly lands on it, you can easily feel it, because your brain is free to sense the change. You know you're doing the Dynamic Relaxer correctly when you find yourself moving without forcing your actions.
- **Rest briefly after each movement.** Again, because your mind as well as your body is engaged in these exercises, it's best to rest for about ten seconds after completing one. Notice any tension in your body, and try to relax that tension before going on.

The Dynamic Relaxer consists of eight simple movements based on t'ai chi, an exercise system developed in China about a thousand years ago. Each should be repeated eight to ten times. The best time to do this exercise is in the morning, before breakfast. However, the routine is an excellent warm-up for competitive sports, as it integrates your nervous system, helping promote peak performance. Get into a relaxed standing pose and begin the first movement:

Movement 1. The Big Arch

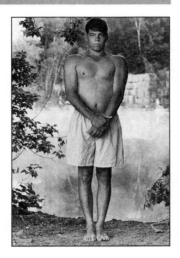

■ Start with your feet together and grasp your left wrist with your right hand.

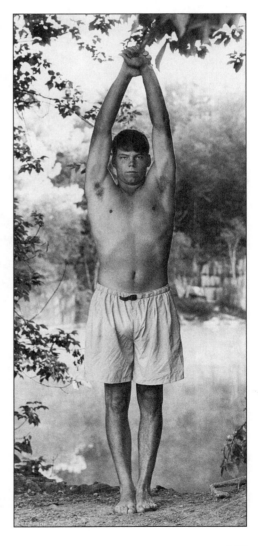

■ As you inhale a deep, slow breath, raise your arms, stretching both hands over your head as high as possible. Hold your breath for a count of two.

■ Exhale slowly and let your arms down.

■ As in all the Dynamic Relaxer movements, if possible inhale and exhale deeply and slowly through your nose. Repeat this arm-raising motion twice to warm up and establish your balance.

■ On your third repetition, raise your heels up off the ground as you extend your arms up, so that when your arms are completely over your head you are balancing on the balls of your feet.

■ Exhale slowly and let your arms down while you lower your heels. Repeat eight to ten times.

Movement 2. The Power Push

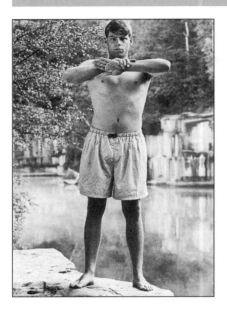

■ After taking a breath or two and letting yourself completely relax, spread your legs so your feet are shoulder-width apart.

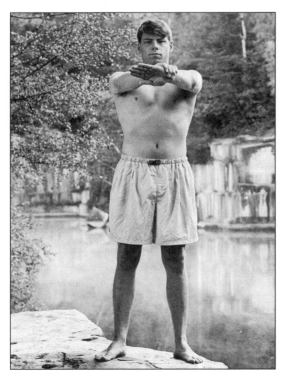

■ Grasp your left wrist with your right hand and hold them at chest level. Taking a breath, push your arms out as far as is comfortable.

■ Exhaling, bring your arms back into your body to the starting position. Repeat eight to ten times.

Movement 3. Kissing the Sky

■ Stand with your feet together. Your arms are at your sides, with your elbows slightly bent and your palms facing backward.

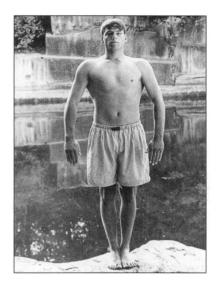

■ As you inhale, arch your head and back so that you're looking straight up, and raise your outstretched arms out to the sides, up to shoulder level, rotating your hands until their palms face the sky.

■ Move slowly to prevent yourself from falling backward. Exhale and return to the starting position. Repeat eight to ten times.

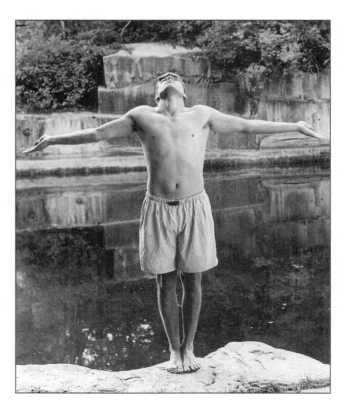

Movement 4. Throwing Open the Window

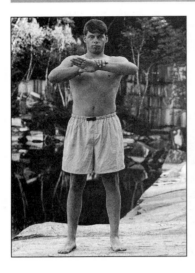

■ Start with your feet shoulder-width apart. Grasp your left wrist with your right hand at chest level, near your left armpit.

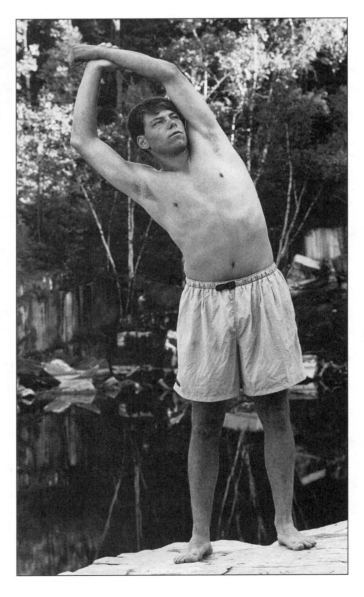

■ As you inhale, raise your hands over your head, bending backward and to the right while you look to the left.

■ Exhale slowly and return to the starting position. Repeat eight to ten times, then switch your stance and repeat on the right side.

Movement 5. Collecting Energy

- Stand with your feet together. Intertwine the fingers of both hands so that the palms of your hands are facing up. Your hands should be at the level of your belly button.

- Inhale and raise your hands up to the level of your chin. As you reach the end of your inhalation, turn your palms down so that they face the ground.

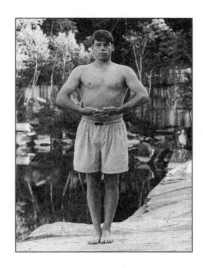

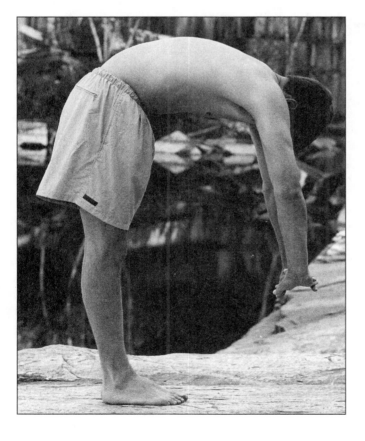

- Exhaling, push your hands down toward the ground. Only bend as far forward as is comfortable. Keep your legs straight.

- Inhale as you turn your palms up and bring your hands back up toward your chin. Repeat eight to ten times, developing a flowing motion of inhaling as you raise your hands and arms, then exhaling as you push your hands toward the ground.

Movement 6. The Big Twist

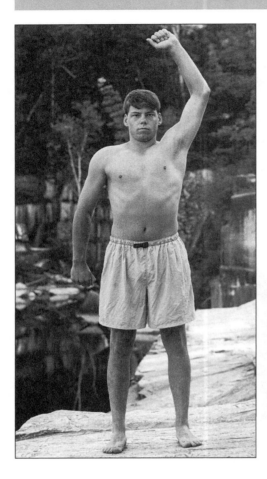

- Start with your feet shoulder-width apart. Make fists with both hands.

- Raise your left arm so that its elbow is bent and at a level even with the top of your head.

- Hold your right arm with its elbow slightly bent and your right hand just below waist level. Inhale a deep breath.

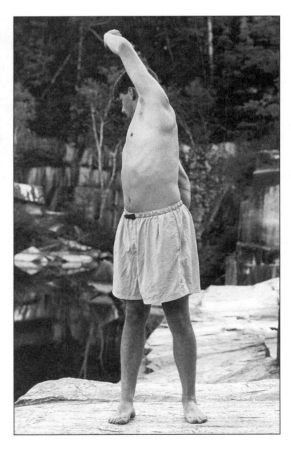

- As you exhale, slowly twist your body and neck to the right and look down toward your buttocks. Repeat eight to ten times.

- Switch your stance and repeat to the left side.

- For more twist, drop the arm that's overhead so that its elbow is bent and level with your shoulders.

Movement 7. The High Dive

- Again, start with your feet shoulder-width apart. Hold your arms straight and slightly in back of you, with your palms facing backward.

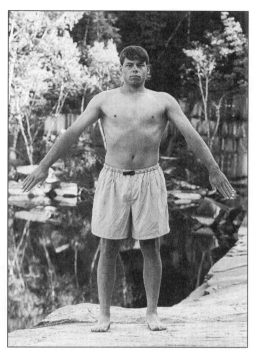

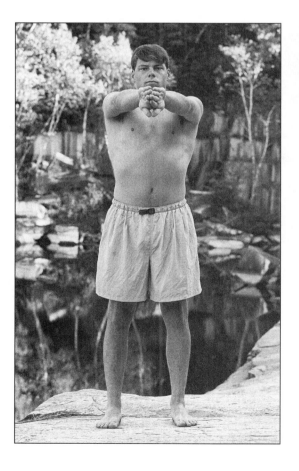

- Taking a long, slow, deep breath, bring your arms in front of you in a smooth arc that brings the backs of your hands together.

- Exhale as you return to the starting position. Repeat eight to ten times.

Movement 8. The Big Reach

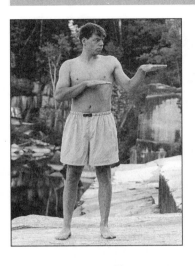

- Again, start with your feet shoulder-width apart.

- Raise your hands up to your chest with the palms of your hands facing the ground.

- Inhale and stretch your hands out to the left, keeping your palms down and your arms parallel to the ground.

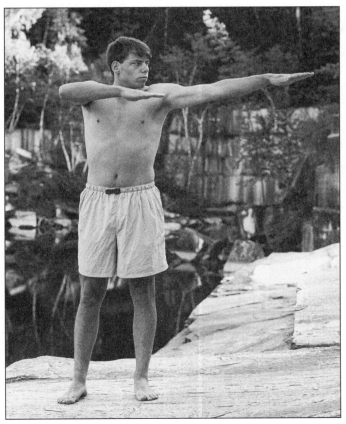

- Stretch out as far as is comfortable while keeping your torso straight.

- Exhale as you return to the starting position. Repeat eight to ten times, and then perform the same movements to the right.

Relax Dynamically in Three Minutes

A great short version of the Dynamic Relaxer is to do four movements each of the Big Arch, the Power Push, Throwing Open the Window (four repetitions each to the right and left), and Collecting Energy. Do this mini-routine throughout the day to keep your spine flexible and your energy high.

My Chiropractor's Advice:

9

BRAIN
BOOSTING

[mental techniques for calming overload]

Joanne's lower back hurt so much it bent her in two. When she came into our clinic for her first appointment, she couldn't raise her head to see over the receptionist's desk. She was crabby and demanding, putting everyone in the office on edge. After two weeks of care she felt much better, and her personality brightened.

Then, one Monday morning, she arrived at the office bent over again, clutching her husband Bob for support as she came through the door. Bob reported that she'd taken a trip to see her mother over the weekend.

"This happens every time she goes up there," he said. "I don't know why she lets that woman treat her the way she does."

It turned out Joanne's mother emotionally mistreated her. The mental anguish generated by the relationship created a tornado of tension in Joanne's body, destroying the spinal alignment we'd been able to establish.

Joanne's back problems were rooted in her thoughts.

Thoughts can stream across our minds like clouds blown by a summer wind. They can also turn heavy, filling our skulls, pounding to get out, demanding our attention.

Beyond the character of your thoughts lies their physical life inside your body. It's in your brain, over the vast fields of cells humming with electrical energy, that thoughts take physical life in the form of tiny energy storms. Every thought is literally a flash of inspiration, a unique pattern of electrical energy.

But a thought's physical life doesn't stop there. The brain is connected directly or indirectly to every cell in your body through nerves. It's as if the cells were restaurant kitchens awaiting commands from the brain on what to prepare. When nerves deliver orders from the brain, the cells go to work, producing fabulous creations that determine how your body works from second to second.

Just as a whiplash-type automobile accident results in nervous system overload by generating physical stresses we can't adapt to, mental stress creates nervous system overload when life's pressures demolish our peace of mind.

It's easy to imagine how this happens when, like Joanne, we're faced with intense emotional situations. Most of the time, however, the thoughts producing nervous system overload are unconscious.

HIDDEN AGENDAS

Unconscious thoughts don't have to be thoughts at all. Many times they are automatic reactions. We react to situations without thinking, as if our minds were giant jukeboxes filled with thousands of records, and the experiences we face cause specific records to play.

For example, when you're learning to drive, it takes all of your attention. Your mind and body are focused on learning this new skill; everything else takes a backseat, so to speak. However, within a remarkably short time your unconscious mind learns all the reactions necessary to drive a car. It makes a new record for your jukebox.

Once this happens, whenever you get in your car your mind starts playing your driving record (please excuse the pun). Your subconscious takes over the chore of driving, freeing your mind to think about important things like whether or not a frozen yogurt would taste good right now.

Soon you can drive for miles without thinking about what you're doing. If you're like my wife, after a while you can apply lipstick in the rearview mirror, feed your child a bagel, and go down the road, all without being too much of a public menace.

Remarkably, once the unconscious takes over a skill, it's much better at directing us than are our conscious thoughts. For example, world-class athletes talk about being "in the zone." At these times the action around them seems to slow and their bodies perform with a will of their own. It's at times like these that athletes achieve their greatest performances.

The shift from premeditated to unconscious action allows us to go through life without having to relearn skills every time we do something. We can make breakfast, eat it, put our clothes on, comb our hair, and perform hundreds of other everyday tasks with our brains "out to lunch." It's thought that we evolved the ability to shift from active to unconscious control of our bodies because it was a quick way to learn survival skills. For example, if our ancestors had to think about how to throw a spear each time they needed to kill something, they would have starved.

But the unconsciousness of life can work against us. Every aspect of health is affected by the unconscious records playing in our minds.

REACTION TIMES

Almost any situation we face in life triggers a reaction in our brains, which then impacts our bodies. The process is illustrated below:

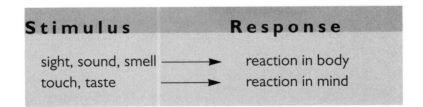

Stimulus		Response
sight, sound, smell	⟶	reaction in body
touch, taste	⟶	reaction in mind

For example, Mike was a fellow chiropractic student. In early November of our first year at chiropractic school, he developed severe low-back pain, seemingly out of nowhere. He couldn't understand why his back started hurting. But in taking a health history, his chiropractor discovered Mike had developed similar attacks during the fall in each of the previous two years. An unconscious pattern, triggered by the time of year, was overloading his nervous system.

INSTANT REPLAY

"Conditioning" is the term scientists use to describe the process whereby a life situation creates a program in our minds that replays itself when triggered by a sight, sound, smell, touch, or taste.

For example, you're running through an airport trying to make a plane that's departing in two minutes. A natural, correct response of your nervous system would be to increase your muscle tension and heart and respiratory rate. Your nervous system is made to adapt you to the world and help you learn as quickly as possible, so the reactions generated by this experience may imprint a program in your nervous system.

Now let's say it's a year after your jog through the airport. You're walking to a plane scheduled to depart in an hour. Something about the situation triggers the program created a year ago. An unconscious reaction takes place, and the same signals from a year ago get sent from your brain into your body. Out of the blue, your body experiences the same muscle tension, pounding heart, and so on as before, even though you have plenty of time to catch the flight. Unconscious conditioning has created nervous system overload.

MIND OVER MATTERS

The good news is that *calm* thoughts create conditioned responses, too. Let's say you take a leisurely vacation to Maui. One afternoon you find yourself in a lounge chair, gazing up into a cloudless blue sky. It seems as if every one of the hundred problems that usually plague you is two thousand miles away. Your body is as limp as cooked linguine. The sun soaks into your skin and releases wonderfully fuzzy feelings of happiness and contentment.

Once back home, if you close your eyes, let your body relax, and think back on that moment of bliss, remembering how the sun felt, the smell of the salt air, and the sound of the rolling waves, your brain will send signals into your body that produce pleasant feelings again.

As we've seen in past chapters, our thoughts have the power to round our shoulders and speed up our hearts. Because they affect the body so profoundly, we need to avoid thoughts that send our nervous systems into overload, generating instead ones that promote tranquillity. If we do, our minds can be the single most powerful tool in eliminating nervous system overload from our lives.

MENTAL ABUSE

I don't think our minds were meant to keep us in a state of nervous system overload. On the contrary, while we tend to let unproductive thought patterns build up over the years, our minds can be wonderful tools to eliminate these old records.

The key to remember is that it's rarely the situations we meet in life that cause our stress reactions. Sometimes, as in the case of running for a plane, circumstances demand that our nervous systems accelerate. Most times, however, it's our *perception* of the situations we find ourselves in that causes the brain to go into overload. That is why a small annoyance can trigger an emotional overreaction that's completely out of proportion to the situation.

Say you're running late to a movie. You throw on your clothes, stuff your keys in your pockets, and "put the pedal to the metal." And then you hit a traffic jam. *Whammo!* The pressure you were already feeling has sensitized your nervous system. All it took was seeing all those brake lights in front of you to send you into overload.

In our office, the forms we hand out to new patients have a space asking them to write in their major health problems. Yesterday a woman wrote, "My children give me migraines." When I asked her about this, she said, "They start screaming and fighting, and within an hour my head is throbbing."

I pointed out that there are many mothers who don't get headaches every time their children misbehave. There must be something else at work. If you get headaches when your children "get on your nerves," what's probably happening is that your children's behavior triggers your brain to run a pattern that creates tight muscles in your neck and on your head. Those tight muscles then pull the bones in your neck out of alignment so that they pinch on the nerves going to your head. It's pinched nerves and the resulting abnormal function of your body—not your children screaming—that create your headaches. If it were possible for you to react to your children's behavior in a different way, so that your brain ran a different program, your nervous system wouldn't be thrown into overload.

As Joan Borysenko notes in her book, *Minding the Body/Mending the Mind:*

> *There are many forces at work in the world that are totally beyond our control and others that we sometimes think are beyond our control but really aren't. To a great extent, our ability to influence our circumstances depends on how we see things. Our beliefs about ourselves and about our own capabilities as well as how we see the world and the forces at play in it all affect what we will find possible.*
>
> *For instance, when you feel overwhelmed by the pressures in your life and you see your own efforts as ineffectual, in all likelihood you will wind up feeling depressed and helpless. Nothing will seem controllable or even worth trying to control. Some of our biggest stresses actually come from our reactions to the smallest, most insignificant events when they threaten our sense of control in one way or another, from the car breaking down just when you have someplace important to go, to your children not listening to you for the tenth time in as many minutes.*

Dr. Wayne Dyer, the popular self-help author, likes to point out that there is no stress in the world, that the world is perfect. He notes that if you squeeze an orange, what comes out is orange juice. If you squeeze a person by putting him in a stressful situation and he responds by becoming angry or nervous, that anger or nervousness is inside of him, not in the situation.

What sends your particular nervous system into overload is very different from what leads mine down that same path. But both of us can decrease the chance of our nervous systems becoming overloaded if we change our thinking. By using some simple mental techniques, we can change the way we perceive stressful situations. Instead of coming up with new ways to deal with every stress in our lives, we can train our nervous systems to handle all stress in a better way.

In the pages ahead you'll learn how to calm your mind and affect the unconscious patterns ingrained in your nervous system. With practice you'll be able to prevent the automatic shift into overload caused by stress.

YOU BE THE JUDGE

The part of your mind most responsible for creating nervous system overload is the one that is forever judging the world. It takes the sights, sounds, smells, and so forth that it receives from the world, or thinks about past or future experiences in terms of those perceptions, and then sets the tone of your muscles to match its evaluation.

The situation in which you are late for a movie and get caught in traffic is a good example. Your mind takes in all those brake lights. It feels you slow to a stop. It notes that you're going to be late. It then makes judgments about the situation that can send your nervous system into overload.

It's difficult to stop your mind from these activities. That's what your mind does. The problem doesn't lie in thinking these thoughts, but in being connected to them so closely.

Most people are so connected to their thoughts that it's impossible to separate themselves from them. It may surprise you that *your thoughts are not you!* It's possible to step back from your thoughts and let them pass by you as if you were watching a parade and they were giant Mickey Mouse balloons.

If you constantly feel connected to tense thoughts, your nervous system becomes like a rope being twisted tighter and tighter. If you consistently separate yourself from your thoughts, you drain tension from your nervous system. This works for unconscious thoughts and reactions as well. When we train our minds to step away from our thoughts, the same inner wisdom that allows top athletes to get "in the zone" starts to work to run our bodies.

The Quiet Mind Technique

Approximate time required: 10 to 20 minutes

The Quiet Mind technique described below is a simplified version of meditation, the practice of which has been shown in hundreds of studies to reduce blood pressure, heart rate, and muscle tension, as well as to decrease anxiety and depression. It is the closest thing to a mental tonic for the nervous system you'll ever find.

In practicing this technique, you'll sit peacefully in a quiet place for ten to twenty minutes with your eyes closed, noticing how your breath moves in and out of your body, counting "one" to yourself every time you breathe out.

As we've seen, breathing is a powerful link between your mind and body. By focusing your attention on it, you give your mind a break. To do the Quiet Mind technique:

1. Find a spot in your house where you'll be able to go at the same time each day to be alone for ten to twenty minutes. Sometimes your bedroom is best, because you can close the door on the rest of the world. You should be able to sit comfortably. If you don't have a suitable chair or couch, try sitting cross-legged on your bed with some pillows propped behind you.

It may be too hectic at home. In that case you can walk or drive to a quiet spot like a park before or after work, or during lunch, to practice the technique.

It's best to practice the Quiet Mind at the same time each day, because you'll be conditioning your nervous system to quiet down just by sitting in the same place at the same time.

The best time is the first thing in the morning, right after your wake-up routine and a few simple stretching exercises (see the Dynamic Relaxer in chapter 8). Your energy will be fresh then, and your muscles limber. However, other times of day will do. If you have trouble sleeping, a bedtime session is a good way to calm down.

2. Once you've found a spot, sit comfortably with your wrists resting on your knees, palms up. Close your eyes.

3. Take a minute to scan your body for tension. Start with a deep inhalation and then give a long sigh as you exhale. As the breath goes out of your body, feel your shoulders drop. Now focus your attention on your head, face, and neck. Are there any tight muscles that could be released? If so, take a deep breath in, and as you breathe out, imagine that your breath is flowing out of the tight spot; feel the muscles in and around the area relax.

Continue scanning your body from the neck down. Focus on the shoulders, arms, chest, upper back, lower back, and belly. Then go down to the legs and feet. As you move through your body, find the tense spots, breathe through them, and let go of any tension. This "body scan" should take only a minute.

4. Now focus on your breath. Notice how it flows into your body, hesitates a bit, and then flows back out. Your natural inclination will probably be to control your breath in some way. For example, you may try to breathe deeper. Don't. Just watch the breath. Let it do whatever it wants. Some forms of meditation teach you to try breathing deeper with each breath. I find that just watching the breath is more relaxing for beginners, as it doesn't impose a "correct" way of breathing that they have to worry about.

If you start to feel anxious, try to let that feeling go. If your anxiety builds, you can take a few deep breaths and stretch your arms up in the air, then go back to watching your breath. If you start to feel really anxious, get up, do some stretching exercises, and try the Quiet Mind technique another time.

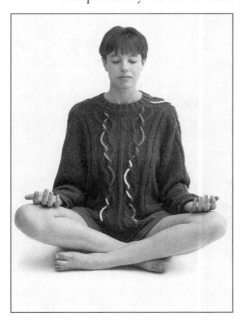

Inside moves. A comfortable position helps your mind relax and focus.

Assuming you don't develop anxiety, as the breath flows out of your body, silently count "one" to yourself. Repeat this process for the next ten to twenty minutes.

As you continue to breathe, you may notice that your breathing gets slower and shallower. Don't be concerned. As your mind quiets, your body quiets too, and it requires less oxygen.

If you don't have ten to twenty minutes, do the Quiet Mind for five. It gets easier with practice. Within two to three weeks you should start to notice that you are feeling more peaceful as nervous system overload melts away.

If you decide that you like training your mind through meditation, there are many excellent books that describe more advanced practices. A classic is *How to Meditate,* by Lawrence LeShan (New York: Bantam Books, 1974).

THE WANDER OF IT ALL

The Quiet Mind is a profoundly simple technique, but it's not as easy to practice as it sounds. For one thing, when you first try it you'll be able to focus on your breath for about as long as it takes to open a bottle of vitamins. Other thoughts—the same ones that constantly go through your mind when you're not concentrating on your breath—will crowd into your head.

You'll be sitting there watching your breath, counting "one" every time you breathe out, and suddenly you'll realize that you're thinking about what you're going to have for lunch, or how your back feels tight, or how you need to call your mother . . . any one of a thousand thoughts will have crept into your mind; you'll notice yourself following them, chasing after them as if you had a net and were chasing butterflies.

You'll realize that you promised yourself that for ten to twenty minutes you were just going to watch your breath go in and out of your body, counting "one" every time you let a breath out. You'll go back to watching and counting. Within two or three breaths you'll catch yourself thinking about filling up the car with gas or wondering if the bathroom needs to be cleaned . . . and so it will go for ten to twenty minutes, with you concentrating on the breath, losing that concentration to a passing thought, chasing the thought, remembering that you should be counting breaths, and going back to counting your breaths until the next thought crosses your mind.

Other things may happen during your Quiet Mind sessions. For example, you may get sleepy, because your body has been trained to go to sleep when you close your eyes and relax. That's why it's best to sit up when you practice.

You may also find yourself feeling anxious. When you quiet your mind, all your worries get a chance to jump onto the stage of your attention. When this happens—and it will—you need to remind yourself that this is a time for letting go instead of holding on. It's one of the few times you can sit back and observe your worries from a distance, choosing to watch them rather than figuring out how to solve them.

You can also get anxious thinking about how bad you are at quieting your mind. "I'll never be good at this," an inner voice might chime. "All I can concentrate on is how good some french fries would taste right now!"

It's natural for ideas to flow across your mind. That's the way your mind works. Don't fight it! Sometimes you'll be able to go for ten seconds before a thought takes you away. Other times it may be a full minute. The length of time between thoughts isn't important. Any Quiet Mind session is a good session!

The Balanced Breather
Approximate time required: 2 to 3 minutes

Sometimes the tight muscles, butterflies in the stomach, racing heart, and other anxious feelings of nervous system overload seem to jump on us from out of the blue. When we feel these sensations, our minds react by increasing our anxiety level even more. At these times it's good to have a technique to break the cycle whereby anxious thoughts create anxious bodies.

The easiest way to do this is with a modification of the Belly Breathing technique you learned in Chapter Seven called the Balanced Breather:

Take a deep breath in and then blow it out completely through your mouth, giving a big sigh of relief. As you breathe out, flatten your belly, squeezing out every last bit of air. Now let the next breath flow in by itself through your nose. Can you feel the belly expand? If not, take another deep breath in and blow it out completely, again flattening your belly. Again let the breath flow in. Breathing this way helps shift your nervous system out of machine-gun mode. Two or three minutes of balanced breathing will usually fend off the anxious symptoms caused by nervous system overload.

SHOCK VALUES

Last night, remote in hand, I was surfing my television's channels. In five minutes I witnessed the following: an actor playing a surgeon reached into what looked like a bloody incision and pulled out a half-digested finger; a news report showed dead soldiers stacked up like firewood in a far-off corner of the world; and in a scene from "Star Trek," photon torpedoes blasted an alien spaceship into interstellar dust.

The assaultive nature of the images and sounds we take in each day is mind-boggling. Bombarded with shocking information, we're like boxers in the fifteenth round who've taken too many punches to the head.

The *volume* of information is staggering, too. It's being poured into us, just like the water we drink. In the Quiet Mind technique, you notice that many of the thoughts prancing across your brain are little bits of commercials, movies, and songs that have been stored in your head! In the Information Age we must wonder, "How much can I take?"

Of all the information sources out there television is the scariest. According to some studies, the television is on in most American homes seven hours a day, and many children watch the tube nearly every minute it's on. That's more time than they spend doing anything else in their lives except sleeping! Much of what they watch is fast-paced and violent, and all of it is artificial. By the time the average child reaches sixteen years of age, he or she has seen approximately 200,000 acts of violence, including 33,000 murders.

In his book *Full Catastrophe Living,* Jon Kabat-Zinn points out that while we plop ourselves down in front of the TV as a way to relax, many times it has just the opposite effect:

The constant agitation of our thinking minds is actually fed and compounded by our diet of TV, radio, newspapers, and movies. We are constantly shoveling into our minds more things to react to; to think, worry, and obsess about, and to remember, as if our own daily lives did not produce enough.

The irony is that we do it to get some respite from our own concerns and preoccupations, to take our mind off our troubles, to entertain ourselves, to carry us away, to help us relax. But it doesn't work that way. Watching television hardly ever promotes physiological relaxation. Its purview is more along the lines of sensory bombardment.

Researchers find it hard to correlate "world stress," as they term the overload of sensory stimulation we receive, with nervous system breakdown. But it makes sense that if your nervous system works best when it is quietly focused on something like your breath, it would probably work worst when being swarmed by sensory stimulation.

RACE COURSE

Life's incredibly fast pace adds to the overload. In my practice, I've found that time stress is one of the biggest barriers to natural living and natural health. Not only does time pressure create stress, it prevents people from allowing their bodies to heal naturally, pushing them toward therapies offering quick fixes that cover up symptoms rather than letting their bodies heal from the inside.

Several months ago an elderly woman came into our clinic complaining of mid-back pain. She had a "hump back" and had been diagnosed with osteoporosis, a condition in which bones become thin and brittle. She said she spent many hours knitting, and that her back hurt constantly, cramping into spasms several times each night.

As I worked on her during her first visit, I let her know that it was going to take several months to make real progress in her spine. The next day she walked into the clinic with a sour look on her face. I greeted her the same way I do most of my patients, saying, "Hi! Good to see you! Ready to get your spine tuned up today?" "My back is still hurting!" she shot back at me, as if in one visit I could erase the twenty to thirty years of degenerative changes in her spine!

Whether their pain began suddenly after an auto accident or developed over years, most patients want it gone *now!*—so they can jump right back into their personal race against the clock.

When patients present this attitude, I ask them if they like to eat spaghetti. Most say yes. I'll ask how long it takes for spaghetti to cook, and they say, "About ten minutes."

"That's right," I'll say. "You know, I'd love for my spaghetti to cook in two minutes, but Mother Nature doesn't care what I think. She's going to take ten minutes to cook my spaghetti. That's because every process in nature requires time. Nature has a timetable for everything. It's the same with your body. Once we get your nervous system functioning correctly, we have to wait for nature to do the healing. That may happen quickly or slowly, but we can't control it. Give nature the time it needs."

If you feel overwhelmed by time pressure, your nervous system acts accordingly. And these days it's easy to feel time pressure. As Kabat-Zinn points out:

> Computers have amplified to such an extent the ability to get paperwork and computations done that, although they are tremendously liberating in some ways, people can find themselves under more pressure than ever to get more done in less time. The expectations of oneself and of others just increase as the technology provides us with the power to do more faster. . . . We will never be out of touch with the world. But will we ever be in touch with ourselves?

How to Stand and Work

Chores such as ironing, washing dishes, or chopping food at a counter increase the stress on your spine. The best way to handle these jobs is to place a box or stool that's about six inches high to the front or side of your body. Put one foot on the box to relieve pressure on your low back. Also, try raising or lowering the surface you're working on, finding the height that keeps your neck and shoulders most relaxed.

TIME INS

How can you protect your nervous system from world stress? Below are four strategies for giving your nervous system a break from sensory bombardment and time pressure. Before you decide you don't have time to try any of these techniques, take a tip attributed to Abraham Lincoln: "Sometimes when there's too much to do, it's best to do nothing."

CHANNEL SURFING WIPEOUT

If it's become a habit for you to spend hours in front of the television, the best way to wean yourself from the tube is to plan your viewing. Don't use the television to baby-sit your brain. Actively choose what you're going to watch, and make sure it's worth sacrificing "real things" like doing some of the activities contained in this book, athletics, playing with the kids, or reading a book. A motivational speaker once noted that if you read one book each week in your chosen field, by the end of one year you'd be in the top five percent of your profession!

Keep a log of your television viewing. For one week, every time you sit in front of the box, write it down. Total the hours at the end of the week, and you may be amazed at how much of your life is spent gazing into a tube that offers only two-dimensional reality.

FLOAT YOUR BOAT

Bathtubs are excellent tools for de-stressing your nervous system. Here's how to turn your tub into a relaxation tank:

- The key to using baths to relax is to decrease input-triggering nervous system activity while increasing relaxing sensations. The best way to separate yourself from the world's normal stimulation is to lock the bathroom door, creating a physical and mental barrier from life's normal pressures.
- Fill the bath with warm water. Heat sedates the mind by increasing blood flow to your muscles, which relaxes them so they send calm messages to your brain.
- Turn down the lights. Try using candles to produce soft, soothing illumination.

- As you decrease the stimulation from light and sound, you'll want to increase sensations from relaxing scents. Today the science of aromatherapy—using scents to affect brain/body function—provides an easy way to calm down. Studies show that scents affect appetite, body temperature, hormone levels, metabolism, stress levels, and sex drive.

Aromatherapists use several plant oils to calm the nervous system. To create a relaxing bath, add six to ten drops of chamomile, lavender, or marjoram "essential oil" to the water as your tub is filling. You can usually buy these concentrated oils from your local health-food store, or you can order them by mail from Aroma Vera, 5901 Rodeo Drive, Los Angeles, CA 90016 (phone 800-669-9514 or 310-280-0407). This company also offers "synergy blends," which are mixtures of oils formulated for their soothing properties.

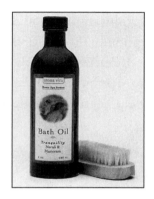

Soothe operator. Aromatic oils provide tub tranquillity.

TAPE DANCE

One of the easiest and quickest ways to achieve relaxation of mind and body is through the new generation of anti-stress cassette recordings. It's best to play these tapes through headphones to get the full benefit of their special use of hypnotic language and acoustics. As you listen, voices guide your thoughts into tranquillity while music soothes your brain. Within ten to thirty minutes the tapes can induce a state of deep relaxation.

Usually priced under ten dollars, these tapes are an inexpensive buffer to Information Age onslaught. If relaxation tapes aren't available at your local health-food store, you can buy my favorite, titled *Deep Relaxation,* from Learning Strategies Corporation, 900 East Wayzata Boulevard, Wayzata, MN 55391 (phone 800-735-8273).

LIGHT SHOW

Push a button and you suddenly see a kaleidoscopic pattern of complex, bright colors dancing before your eyes while rhythmic sounds pulse in your ears. You're connected to a "light-and sound" machine. These high-tech answers to stress guide your brain's activity into a pattern of relaxation or other states, such as increased creativity or learning ability. Priced from around $150, light-and-sound machines are available from Tools for Exploration, 4460 Redwood Highway, Suite 2, San Rafael, CA 94903 (phone 800-456-9887 or 415-499-9047).

Perhaps someday the world outside ourselves will be more conducive to nervous system tranquillity. Until then, the techniques listed above can help keep world stress at a distance.

My Chiropractor's Advice:

10

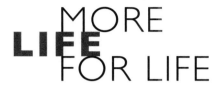

MORE
LIFE
FOR LIFE

[eliminating nervous system overload forever]

The exercises and other techniques in this book will, if practiced consistently, create more health in your life.

This approach, which builds health from the inside out, is very different from that of conventional medicine, which wants to take responsibility for your health. You go to the doctor, and he or she "fixes" you. Chiropractic shifts the responsibility for your health to where it belongs— on your back, so to speak.

Virtually all of our patients first come to our office because they are in pain. But then we try to teach them that true health is not the absence of pain or other symptoms, but a body and mind functioning at the very highest level possible.

For example, I'll tell patients, "If you wanted to win an Olympic gold medal in running, could you make the Olympic team by running for five minutes a week? When you want your body to do something better, you have to train it. If you want your nervous system to work better, you have to train it, too."

Chiropractors work wonders, but the people coming into our clinics often bring problems they've had for many years, problems that only recently began producing noticeable symptoms. Correcting the underlying problems takes work, but it can be fun.

TRAINING TABLE

You're about to develop a training program for achieving 100 percent nervous system function. Using the chart on pages 181–85, you'll follow a three-step process.

First you'll identify the exercises and techniques best suited to your current condition. Next you'll review your schedule and find time to use this book's ideas. Finally you'll write a schedule for *this week* so you can start training.

In developing a personal training program, first consider if you are currently in pain. What part or parts of your body hurt the worst?

NIGHTMARE NECK

If you're dealing with neck pain and/or headaches your training should emphasize chapter 5's neck pain relief routine. If your chiropractor has given you this book, follow his or her directions in doing the exercises. If not, here are some guidelines:

- If you are in too much pain to sleep or otherwise rest comfortably, or if your pain does not become progressively better after doing the exercises in this book several times, consult a chiropractor, as your symptoms most likely need professional help.
- **Do not do any exercise that causes you pain.** Typically, you'll be able to do all the exercises if you're gentle with yourself. Do very small movements at first, increasing them until you reach a pain threshold, then back off. **Again, as soon as you feel pain, decrease your movements.**

Pushing yourself into the pain zone when exercising is counterproductive. When your body sends pain signals to the brain, the brain responds by tightening muscles in that area of the body. So if your neck is hurting and you really stretch it, the neck muscles usually become tighter.

- In general, you should follow the number of repetitions given with each exercise. If you enjoy a particular exercise, increase the number of repetitions as your neck pain begins to fade.
- If you find that certain exercises relieve your pain symptoms better than others, by all means spend more time on them. Likewise, leave out any exercises that aggravate your condition.
- Breathing deeply and slowly is as important when doing the exercises as are the exercises themselves. Let your breathing help relax your muscles.

If headaches are your main problem, do the Trigger Fingers technique two times each day, in the morning and at night before bed. Do the technique before your neck exercises to make them more effective.

Also helpful if you're suffering from headaches and/or neck pain are the relaxation techniques in chapter 9. Practicing the Quiet Mind routine can often give you a different perspective on your pain, providing some distance from it, making it more manageable.

If your neck pain is not accompanied by headaches, concentrate on the stretching exercises and the self-massage technique. Perform self-massage on your neck and shoulders at least three times a day at work to help relieve the strain of sitting at a desk. Take a break from your chores every hour or two to stretch and massage. This need only take two or three minutes, and can coincide with bathroom breaks and mealtimes so that you don't feel time pressure.

The heat of a bath containing a de-stressing essential oil will help relax your neck muscles, and when used in conjunction with self-massage, it can help break the spasm-pain-spasm cycle at the root of many neck pains. In addition, the natural relaxants described in chapter 7, including valerian and chamomile, will help take the edge off of your pain.

BACK BITTEN

If your back hurts, concentrate on the back pain relief program in chapter 6. All the advice given above for doing the neck pain relief exercises applies to your back as well. Be as gentle with your back as possible when doing the exercises, and de-stress as often as you can with relaxing baths and the other calming techniques in chapter 9.

If your job requires lifting, twisting, or other motions that make your back hurt, talk to your supervisor about doing light-duty work until your back is feeling better. The same advice goes for household chores, including lifting small children.

Many people with back pain try to live with it, going about their normal daily routines, and end up severely injuring themselves. Most people require back operations only after they've had many warning signs from their backs, but they've chosen to ignore them. One day the dam breaks, and they wind up under the knife because areas of their bodies that withstand a great deal of punishment have degenerated beyond the point of rehabilitation.

Although low-back pain may come and go, most low-back problems *don't improve with time, but only with care.*

Your back may recuperate faster if you wear a back brace while driving and doing other activities. The best braces are the big black ones designed **for** manual laborers. They are available in mass merchandise-type stores such as K mart and Wal-mart, special orthopedic supply stores, or through your chiropractor. Wrap the brace snugly around your back, but not so tightly that it interferes with your breathing.

Thinner back braces that you wear under your clothes are also available. Offering less support, they nonetheless restrict your back so that you don't move foolishly, and can be beneficial.

While back braces are helpful for relieving pain and giving you a sense of security, don't rely on one for long; they may give you the feeling that your back isn't really hurt. If you need a brace to feel good, that's not the case.

SOOTHING THE MINDS THAT BIND US

Obviously, if you're feeling overwhelmed by anxiety or depression, it's best to seek a professional mental health counselor or therapist. But for mild bouts of these common mental difficulties, you'll want to exercise your body and mind. The Dynamic Relaxer exercise and the Quiet Mind technique should be cornerstones of your self rehabilitation, as well as chapter 7's breathing exercises, nerve herbs, and vitamins.

Regular aerobic exercise can also be a powerful personal tool for combating feelings of anxiousness and depression. At the risk of sounding incredibly naive, if we could only take a brisk walk every night with a friend with whom we could discuss our problems, many of our anxious or depressed thoughts would disappear.

ABOVE AND BEYOND

In time, you should reach a point in your health quest where getting out of pain isn't your main concern. If you've had neck, headache, or back problems for a long time, you'll want to keep doing your favorite pain-relief exercises every day. But you'll also want to practice other techniques to achieve higher health levels.

A good place to start is at the table. Nutrition so powerfully affects your nervous system that you'll want to get this piece of the health puzzle into place as quickly as possible. Don't try to change all your eating habits overnight. Try a cleansing diet and then incorporate as many of the suggestions in chapter 7 as are comfortable.

You'll also need to work on your breathing, and it's a great time to try the wake-up routine in chapter 4. If you're not participating in an aerobic activity such as running, walking, swimming, or bicycling, now is an excellent time to start. Get your heart pumping for at least twenty minutes, three times each week. Any of these changes will boost your health dramatically.

If you work at a desk, or notice that your shoulders have rounded and your head has dropped over the years, you'll find the Perfect Posture Program in chapter 5 especially helpful. With daily practice you should notice postural changes within six to eight weeks. Even doing one or two of the exercises at your desk throughout the day will help prevent your neck and shoulders from becoming stiff and sore.

Once your low back stops hurting, you'll want to move on to the Pelvic Power routine in chapter 6. The energy these exercises generate inside your pelvis will help rejuvenate every inch of you, and you may find sexual activities take on a new excitement.

Also rejuvenating are chapter 8's Neurological Flush and Dynamic Relaxer exercises. Use them as part of a morning wake-up ritual or as a warm-up before athletic or aerobic activities.

Optimally, your personal program will comprise the following:

- **a morning wake-up routine that includes stretching exercises**
- **eating for energy**
- **supplementing your diet with herbs and vitamins that fuel peak nervous system function**
- **practicing breathing for energy whenever possible**
- **a regular aerobic conditioning program**
- **practicing the Quiet Mind technique ten to twenty minutes each day**

Sound like a lot? Actually, you can do all this in about an hour, spread throughout your fourteen-hour day. Using the table on pages 181–85, pick activities and write times during your day to train.

The key is to make health a lifestyle. You may not be able to cram more activities into your present life. Instead, start replacing some of the things you're doing now with the activities described in this book. If you do, there's no way health can keep away from you.

SEARCH PARTY

Throughout this book I've stressed the importance of working with a chiropractor in order to achieve the best and fastest results. I'm sometimes asked by patients who are moving to another state, "How can I find a good chiropractor?" I think a better question might be "How do I find a chiropractor who's right for me?"

Virtually all chiropractors are great—for some people. I've had patients come to me after treatment by another chiropractor and tell me, "You just don't work on me like Dr. Smith." They'll ask if I can do this or that, and while I try to give them the same treatment as their last doctor, often I'm not up to the task. The reason is that while the study of chiropractic is a science, the practice of chiropractic is an art.

No two chiropractors work on your body the same way, because chiropractic involves a personal relationship between doctor and patient.

With that in mind, here are some guidelines for choosing a chiropractor with whom you'll feel comfortable:

- Find a chiropractor by asking your friends for a referral. You'll be surprised how many of your friends are already getting their spines checked on a regular basis. Chances are, if they've been treated with respect and caring, you will be too.
- Once you've received a referral to a chiropractor, call the doctor's office and ask if he or she will consult with you for a small fee or at no charge. It's standard practice for chiropractors to consult with prospective patients before examining them or doing other procedures. If the doctor thinks your condition requires another physician's treatment, she or he can refer appropriately. Even if you are referred to another type of doctor, remember that only a chiropractor is trained to get your nervous system functioning perfectly. Though you may have symptoms requiring nonchiropractic attention, you are always better off, no matter what condition you may have, if your nervous system is functioning properly.
- Don't be alarmed if the chiropractor wants to take X rays of your spine. Many want pictures of your neck and back before beginning treatment. This is usually a good idea. The information gained from X rays can be of enormous help in getting your spine into optimum condition.
- Your chiropractor should make your care affordable. Often patients require several months of treatment to correct spinal problems. Though most insurance plans cover chiropractic, they often only pay for a limited number of visits. This may be enough to get you out of pain, but you may well need more care to correct your problem. If this is your case, your chiropractor should make financial arrangements with you that fit your budget. This goes for your entire family. Often children need chiropractic care. The need goes undetected because they either haven't developed symptoms or the medical doctors treating their symptoms aren't

aware of how well chiropractic can help in alleviating many common childhood problems. Some responding particularly well include chronic ear and bronchial infections, sinus troubles, colic, asthma, allergies, and bedwetting.

• Finally, if you feel uncomfortable with your spinal specialist, discuss your concerns with him or her. Often the chiropractor can change treatment methods to suit your individual needs.

Regarding this last item, if you do have an unpleasant experience with a chiropractor, don't give up on chiropractic! It amazes me how people will try one medical doctor after another, but a person who has a single bad experience with one chiropractor might never try chiropractic again. There's a chiropractor out there just right for you and your family.

BALANCING ACT

Nervous system overload is an epidemic in our society. It seems as if the physical, mental, emotional, and chemical stresses of today's world are only getting worse. However, I believe we have the knowledge and resources to live the healthiest lives ever. We can solve many of our common health problems by fixing their root cause.

By eliminating the interference between the intelligence that runs our bodies and our bodies themselves, we can experience vibrant, vital health.

I hope the seeds within these pages help you grow more health in your life. They are offered with appreciation and love.

My Chiropractor's Advice:

Total Nerve Flow in Three Easy Steps

Step 1

Choose the exercises and other techniques for your personal program

CHAPTER 4

□ The Sunny Side Wake-Up Routine

CHAPTER 5

Neck Pain Relief

□ Shoulder Shrug
□ Shoulder Shrug, Part 2
□ The Reader
□ Trigger Fingers
□ Self-Massage

The Perfect Posture Program

□ The Ball Bearing
□ The Back Loop
□ The Wall Slide
□ The Chest Breath
□ The Seagull
□ The Turtle/Turtle, Part 2

CHAPTER 6

Back Pain Relief

□ The Knee Pull
□ The Deep Tilt
□ The Side-to-Side
□ The Bicycle
□ The Back Builder
□ Abdominal Crunches

Pelvic Power

- ☐ The Sacral Sit-Back
- ☐ The Roundhouse
- ☐ The Pump

CHAPTER 7

Eating for Energy

- ☐ Three-Day Cleansing Diet
- ☐ Fruit for Breakfast
- ☐ Dinner Before Six
- ☐ Proper Food Combining
- ☐ Decreased Protein

Breathing for Energy

- ☐ Belly Breathing
- ☐ The 1-4-2 Breath
- ☐ The Sixty-Second Exhaler

Vitamin and Herb Supplementation

- ☐ beta-carotene
- ☐ vitamin B complex
- ☐ vitamin C
- ☐ vitamin E
- ☐ ginkgo biloba
- ☐ ginseng
- ☐ valerian
- ☐ chamomile

CHAPTER 8

- ☐ The Neurological Flush
- ☐ The Dynamic Relaxer

CHAPTER 9

- ☐ The Quiet Mind Technique
- ☐ The Balanced Breather
- ☐ Edited television viewing
- ☐ Relaxing essential oil baths
- ☐ Relaxation tapes
- ☐ Sound-and-light machines

Step 2

Identify available training time

Morning

- ☐ Before breakfast
- ☐ During morning commute to work
- ☐ Bathroom breaks
- ☐ Work breaks

Afternoon

- ☐ Lunch
- ☐ Bathroom breaks
- ☐ Work breaks

Evening

- ☐ During evening commute from work
- ☐ Before dinner
- ☐ At the dinner table
- ☐ During an evening bath
- ☐ While watching television
- ☐ In bed, before going to sleep

Step 3

Design your training schedule

Monday

Morning _____

Afternoon _____

Evening _____

Tuesday

Morning _____

Afternoon _____

Evening _____

Wednesday

Morning _____

Afternoon _____

Evening _____

Thursday

Morning _____

Afternoon _____

Evening _____

Friday

    Morning ————————————————————————

    Afternoon ————————————————————————

    Evening ————————————————————————

Saturday

    Morning ————————————————————————

    Afternoon ————————————————————————

    Evening ————————————————————————

Sunday

    Morning ————————————————————————

    Afternoon ————————————————————————

    Evening ————————————————————————

My Chiropractor's Advice:

APPENDIX

{pain relief for carpal tunnel syndrome and arthritis}

CARPAL TUNNEL SYNDROME

What causes wrist pain? The most common culprit is pinched nerves in the hands, wrists, or arms.

Your wrists contain eight bones. If these bones get out of proper alignment, they can pinch nerves in the wrists, causing pain, numbness, and tingling. Inflammation or swelling often follows, so that muscles and ligaments in the wrists and arms become constantly irritated. Pinched nerves are usually brought on by activity, especially repetitive tasks, such as cutting hair, typing at a computer, or playing the piano. Often the wrist of the hand that uses the computer's "mouse" will be particularly sore after a long day.

What can you do about pinched nerves in your wrist?

Take action. Don't wait. Wrist problems are usually easy to manage if you address them when you first notice discomfort. If you let the problem go on for months or years, you run the risk of wrist surgery.

The following is a home treatment program to help keep your wrists pain free.

Superwrist Program

Stretching Exercises

Stretching the muscles involved will relieve stress from your wrists, helping them heal. Do the following exercises in the morning, before starting your job, and throughout the day to keep your wrists loose and flexible.

The Power Push

Start by putting your hands together in a prayer position. Turn your hands so that your fingers are pointing toward your chest. Now, keeping your hands pressed together, slowly spread your fingers and push your hands away from your body. Feel a good stretch in the muscles on the underside of your wrists. Taking deep, slow breaths, hold this position for 15 seconds. Every time you exhale, try to gently push your hands out a bit, getting a little more stretch.

The Palm Stretch

Spread your hands, palms up, resting on your knees. (Your thumbs and "pinky" finger should be as far apart as possible.) Slowly bring your thumb and pinky together, then spread them apart. Feel your thumb stretch away from your pinky finger on each repetition. You should feel a good stretch across the palms of your hands. Do fifteen repetitions.

The Thumb Tuck

Extend your hand as if you were going to shake hands. Tuck your thumb toward the palm of your hand, and wrap your fingers around the thumb. Bend your wrists forward, so that the muscles connecting your thumbs to your wrists and forearms get a good stretch. Do this motion slowly. If you feel pain at some point during the stretch, STOP! You don't want to cause yourself pain. As soon as you feel pain, stop the motion and let the wrist relax, then slowly stretch again to the point of pain. Do fifteen repetitions.

Strengthening Exercises

Strengthening your wrist will help keep the muscles, ligaments and carpal bones in top shape. If you do repetitive-motion work each day, such as typing or cutting hair, you should train the muscles of your wrist on a daily basis. To do this exercise you need to obtain a three-pound barbell (for women) or a five-pound barbell (for men) from a sporting goods store. (This is a general guideline. I realize some women are as strong or stronger than men.)

- Hold the barbell in your right hand so that your wrist is straight, palms up, parallel to the floor. Lift the weight up, bending your wrist toward your arm, and then let it back down to the starting position. Your arm should remain steady; movement should be in the wrist. Repeat 10 times to start.

- Switch the barbell to the left hand and repeat.

- Now take the barbell in your right hand again and assume the starting position, with the weight parallel to the floor and your palm facing down. Drop the barbell toward the floor and then raise it back up, again, moving just your wrist while your arm remains steady.

- Switch the barbell to the left hand and repeat.

- Do the four wrist strengthening exercises every day. Add five repetitions each week, building up to thirty-five repetitions. Once you're able to easily do thirty-five repetitions with no pain or soreness, decrease the number of times you do this exercise to three times each week to maintain muscle tone.

Note: If you have extremely small wrists, start with a two-pound barbell. If you have large wrists, start with a five-pound weight.

NUTRITIONAL SUPPLEMENTATION

Studies show that supplementing your diet with vitamin B complex and a vitamin B_6 supplement helps heal your wrists.

Take one 100 mg vitamin B complex and one vitamin B_6 supplement each day for one to three months or until your wrist pain goes away. Continue with a B complex supplement as part of your regular diet thereafter.

USING SUPPORTS

While your wrists are healing, it's good to give them as much rest as possible. Since you still need to work, I recommend using wrist braces until your pain fades. Wrist braces are available from most pharmacies. You'll need two types. Wear a soft, elastic brace while working and driving. Don't wear the brace when you are just relaxing (for example, when you're sitting watching a movie).

At night you should wear a cook-up wrist splint, so named because a metal stay within the brace "cocks" your wrist up and relieves nerve pressure in the wrist while you sleep.

Continue wearing the night brace until you can wake up in the morning without any wrist pain. Continue wearing the soft braces until you can work without pain.

HEAT THERAPY

Applying heat to the wrists will help bring more blood to them, promoting healing.

Obtain a gel-type hot pack. These are available for about five dollars from most pharmacies. Heat the pack and wrap it in a moist dishtowel or dry paper towel. Wrap the pack/towel over your wrist and secure it into place with an elastic bandage. Be sure the pack isn't too hot; if it feels uncomfortably warm, let it cool for a few minutes before wrapping it around the wrist. Leave on for ten minutes. Try to do this once a day. An excellent time is right before going to bed at night.

THE BEST WAY TO DEAL WITH WRIST PROBLEMS: CHIROPRACTIC CARE

You will achieve much quicker results with the program outlined above if you receive chiropractic care for your wrist problems. Chiropractic has an outstanding record in treating wrist, elbow, and shoulder problems. Your chiropractor will examine your neck, shoulders, elbows, and wrists, pinpointing trouble spots where misaligned bones are pinching on nerves. Once this nerve pressure is relieved, your wrists should heal relatively quickly.

Arthiritis Pain Relief Program

One in seven Americans must cope with some kind of arthritis. Usually this involves taking nonsteroidal anti-inflammatory drugs, such as aspirin, ibuprofen, or naproxen. These drugs can cause nasty side effects, such as internal bleeding. The following is a better, natural way for handling arthritis, one that not only decreases pain but in some cases can reverse some of the damage caused by the disease.

STEP ONE: REGULAR CHIROPRACTIC ADJUSTMENTS

Adjustments to the spine and other areas of your body keep joints moving freely, preventing them from "locking up." This helps prevent swelling, increases range of motion, and ensures that the joints receive proper nerve and blood flow. Adjustments can be the single best way to make sure joints don't deteriorate.

STEP TWO: VITAMIN SUPPLEMENTATION

A recent study of 640 people at Boston University found that people taking high doses of vitamin C were three times less likely to suffer progression of arthritis than those not taking the supplements. Dosage: Take 500 mg of vitamin C three times a day. Vitamin E has been shown to have similar effects to vitamin C. Dosage: Take 400 IUs of vitamin E each day.

STEP THREE: OTHER SUPPLEMENTS

Recent research indicates that glucosamine supplements, available at health stores, reduce pain as effectively as ibuprofen, with fewer side effects. Some promising studies show taking glucosamine may even slow down and reverse cartilage damage in arthritic joints. Don't expect instant relief. You need to take glucosamine daily for four to eight weeks before seeing results. Dosage: Take 1 g of glucosamine daily.

GLA, or gamma-linolenic acid, is another substance that experts believe will help arthritic joints heal. Dosage: Take 500 mg of Evening Primrose Oil, which contains GLA, each day.

STEP FOUR: LEARN TO DO ACUPRESSURE ON YOURSELF

Again, studies show acupressure with help relieve your arthritic pain. Buy the book *Arthritis Relief at Your Fingertips* by Michael Reed Gach (Warner Books, 1988). It describes dozens of techniques for relieving arthritis symptoms.

STEP FIVE: START USING CREAMS CONTAINING CAPSAICIN

Capsaicin is the active ingredient in cayenne pepper. It's been shown to block the transmission of pain inside nerve fibers and works well to help ease the pain of stiff, aching joints. Capsaicin creams are available at health food stores and pharmacies. Apply the cream to your affected joints as often as needed.

STEP SIX: EXERCISE

The worst thing an arthritis sufferer can do is become sedentary. Moving and stretching is essential if you want to keep your joints healthy. Some promising new studies show that the ancient Oriental exercise system of Tai Chi, using slow stretching movements combined with deep breathing, is excellent for rejuvenating aging joints. The Dynamic Relaxer exercise found in chapter eight is based on Tai Chi. Do the complete routine every day for arthritis of the feet, knees, hips, spine, neck, shoulders, and hands.

Joint degeneration in the fingers and hands is common. The Palm Stretch, Power Push, and Thumb Tuck exercises included in the Superwrist Program are excellent for keeping hands loose and limber.

Walking, swimming, and bicycling are all good activities to keep joints mobile. Water aerobics classes are even better. Using hot tubs can be comforting, as can soaking in a warm bath for at least twenty minutes at home.

STEP SEVEN: EAT WELL/KEEP YOUR WEIGHT DOWN

A low-fat, mostly vegetarian diet is the best way to eat if you have arthritis. Cut out red meat. Eat lots of leafy green vegetables. Such a diet will improve your overall health while decreasing the inflammation in your joints.

INDEX